50

√

412

# TREATING THE BRAIN

# TREATING THE BRAIN

*What the Best Doctors Know*

Dr. Walter G. Bradley

DANA
PRESS

New York • Washington, D.C.

THE DANA FOUNDATION
745 Fifth Avenue, Suite 900
New York, NY 10151

Dana Press
The Dana Center
900 15th Street NW
Washington, DC 20005

DANA is a federally registered trademark.

ISBN-13: 978-1-932594-46-1

This publication is designed to provide accurate and authoritative information in regard to the subject matter covered. It is sold with the understanding that the publisher is not engaged in rendering professional services. If professional advice or other expert assistance is required, the services of a competent professional person should be sought.

Library of Congress Cataloging-in-Publication Data:
    Bradley, W. G. (Walter George)
        Treating the brain : what the best doctors know / Walter G. Bradley.
        p. cm.
    Includes bibliographical references.
    ISBN 978-1-932594-46-1 (alk. paper)
        1. Neurology—Popular works. 2. Brain—Diseases—Popular works. I. Title.
RC346.B665 2009
616.8—dc22
                    2009020021

Cover design by Debbie Mioduszewski
Interior design by William Stilwell
Art direction by Kenneth Krattenmaker
Illustrations by Kathryn Born

Printed in the United States of America

www.dana.org

# CONTENTS

# ILLUSTRATIONS

# Acknowledgments

This book would not have been started without the education that I have received from my patients over the last fifty years. Their willingness, despite their suffering, to talk to me and to listen to what I had to say in return is the bedrock on which this book is founded. I thank them for their confidence in me, for their openness and for their friendship.

It would not have been completed without the support and encouragement of my wife, Jeanne Baker, who read several drafts with her eagle eye and helped me to see better ways to present my ideas.

Many others have contributed to the final manuscript and I cannot thank them enough for making this a better book. My agent, Albert LaFarge provided insights into writing a popular medical book that were invaluable and led me through the difficult path of bringing this work to the public. Kara Baskin provided me with invaluable help in polishing the manuscript and bringing it to the level of presenting it to the publisher. I particularly want to thank Jane Nevins, vice president of The Dana Foundation and editor in chief of Dana Press, not only for accepting the manuscript for publication but especially for her many insightful suggestions of how to improve each and every chapter.

Many other colleagues, too numerous to mention, have read some of the chapters and made suggestions. Whether or not I was able to adopt your suggestions, I greatly appreciate all your comments.

Walter Bradley DM FRCP
Miami, May 2009

## Chapter 1

# The Human Brain, Complex and Fascinating

We take our brains for granted. We often forget that this amazing three pounds of soft Jell-O is responsible for all our interactions with our environment. Our brains make us the thinking, feeling, reasoning human beings that we are. But when a problem develops in the brain, we want to know *everything* about it. Some problems with the brain, such as a stroke, make us dramatically aware that something is wrong. Others, like Alzheimer's disease, creep up on us. Either way, treatment by a neurologist may come into your life or the life of someone you care about, and that's what this book is about.

Patients and their loved ones want to understand the brain diseases that they suffer from, and they want to know what they are likely to face as they deal with it. Doctors should provide everyone involved with information about the cause of a disease and its treatment. Informed patients and families handle brain conditions better and are more likely to follow their doctors' treatment recommendations. The initial dialogue about the disease, its diagnosis, and its treatment is the most important part of establishing a good doctor-patient relationship. When facing any disease, patients and their families want to know what is going to happen. However, doctors are often reluctant to talk about the prognosis, particularly to the patient. Nowhere is this truer than in the field of neurological diseases.

Forty years ago, when I became a neurologist, people outside medicine had very little access to information about neurological diseases, other than through their doctor. Nowadays, numerous support organizations representing specific diseases—such as the Muscular Dystrophy Association, the ALS Association, and the Alzheimer's Association—provide information for patients and families through brochures and Web sites. We are all part of the Information Age, and most patients have access to the resources of the World Wide Web.

Patients sometimes come to me having made their own diagnoses based on information they found online. Some physicians feel intimidated by this, but I welcome the way that information empowers the patient. Information from the Web has its problems, however. So much of what patients find online is inaccurate, and much of it comes from companies that have a product to sell. Even if the information is accurate, patients often do not have enough background knowledge to interpret a complex medical diagnosis and treatment plan.

This book is intended to make neurology understandable to the layman. It covers some of the most common neurological conditions, how they are diagnosed and treated, and their likely outcomes. It is particularly intended for readers without medical training and people who are worried about neurological diseases. But I hope that this book will interest many other people in what I like to call the Last Frontier—namely, the brain—which can surprise and amaze us even when it's in trouble. I also hope that this book might even stimulate a few medical students to go into the most fascinating medical subspecialty: neurology.

I have included many stories about patients in this book. Patients make up a large part of the life of a physician, even for someone who is involved in a good deal of research and administration, as I am. Much of our current knowledge about the normal and abnormal function of the nervous system comes from stories of individual patients. That is why we need more than just neuroscientists doing research on the nervous system, and more than just neurologists caring for patients. We need neurologist-neuroscientists, who diagnose the patient's problem, investigate it in the laboratory, and do research to understand the disease and how it affects the normal functioning of the brain. Generally neurologist-neuroscientists are academic neurologists who also teach medical students and young doctors in training.

When teaching, I use patient vignettes to drive home significant "clinical pearls," tidbits that the young doctors will remember for the rest of their careers. I also use patient stories to highlight how much our knowledge has advanced in just the few short decades of my career. The stories that I write about in this book are all derived from people I have met over the years. Some of the details have been changed to maintain patient privacy. At times I have combined the stories of two patients for conciseness, and in some places I have constructed dialogue to make the narrative livelier. However, I have tried to maintain the spirit of each person's true story.

If you or a loved one has a neurological problem, then your interest in the brain and neurology is very personal. You want to know as much as possible about your particular condition—how the neurologist made the diagnosis and whether it was correct, the latest information about the condition and how it is treated, and what is going to happen to you. Most of all, you want reassurance that you are being cared for in the best possible fashion by an experienced and compassionate neurologist.

In these pages, I will present enough information for someone who wants to know about each condition, whether it is you or a loved one who has been diagnosed with a neurological disease. I will try to make everything understandable and help you though the morass of detail and long medical terms. I will try to present the good and the bad, but I will always leave you with hope—hope that comes from a clearer understanding about the disease and current treatments, and hope that comes from ongoing research.

Before we embark on our journey through the common neurological diseases in Chapters 2 through 12, you need to have a basic understanding of the anatomy and physiology of the brain. If you do not have this basic knowledge, continue reading this chapter. If you are already knowledgeable about how the brain works but want to look deeper, Appendix A is intended for you.

The brain is the finely tuned instrument that allows us to accomplish amazing feats of mental and physical agility. In good health, we need to respect and protect the brain if we expect it to do everything that we ask of it. That means we must avoid head injuries and refrain from exposing our brains to poisons like excessive amounts of alcohol. When the nervous system is afflicted by an illness, we need to understand what caused the disease and how the nervous system is responding. In the remainder of this chapter, I will tell you much of what we know about the various parts of the nervous system. I will also discuss how patients and their diseases have helped us understand what those parts do. A great deal of this knowledge has come from the study of patients with strokes and penetrating head injuries.

But first, let me set out some basic facts. The human brain has about 100 billion ($10^{11}$) neurons. Each neuron is able to signal many other neurons through connections called synapses. In the outer layer (cerebral cortex) of the human brain, each neuron makes contact with about ten thousand other neurons, and the human cortex has about 0.15 quadrillion ($1.5 \times 10^{13}$) synapses. That's an enormous amount of "wiring." The human cerebral cortex works like an enormously complex computer that can theoretically perform up to $2 \times 10^{16}$ calculations per second.

Since we clearly do not work this fast when doing mathematical calculations, you might ask, Do we fully use the capacity of our brains? The answer is yes, but we are unaware of 90 percent of what our brains are doing. Yet our brain's neurons and synapses allow us to be self-aware, to think, to feel, and—for some of us—to have the agility of a ballet dancer or professional athlete. The brain, the spinal cord, and the peripheral nerves, which collectively are termed the nervous system, provide us with amazing powers.

## The Cerebral Cortex

The cerebral cortex is the most complex and most highly developed part of the brain, as well as the most fascinating. It is the seat of memories, judgment, thought, creativity, free will, and the intellect. Let me tell you about just a few of the seemingly limitless abilities of the human cerebral cortex.

A clerk in one of my hospitals is able to multiply two sets of six-figure numbers in his head. He does this in less time than it takes me to use a calculator to confirm that he is correct. He is equally fast and accurate with the division of ten-figure numbers by five-figure numbers. I have asked him how he does this, and all he can say is, "I just see the numbers in my mind, and the answer is there." Mathematical activity is carried out in the cerebral cortex at the junction between the left temporal and parietal lobes of the brain. Perhaps this man has more synapses in that area than a "normal" person.

In Oliver Sacks's book *The Man Who Mistook His Wife for a Hat*, twin idiot savants correctly count the total number of matchsticks that fall from a matchbox to the floor. Although the twins were mentally disabled, their brains must have had an astounding ability to access the power of their visual association areas.

You must know people who have the habit of finishing sentences for someone they are talking with. Presumably they do this by hearing the first part of what the person is saying, forecasting what he is going to say next—even more quickly than the speaker is talking—and then saying it before the speaker is able to do so. Quite a feat!

Intuition is something that some people believe in and others don't. Women are said to be more intuitive than men. Intuition is a prediction or insight that comes about when we take in complex information and process it in our brains. The intuition may be about how a person is feeling or an event that is going to happen. Though we do not know how we came to the prediction, we say that we have a "funny feeling" about it. Intuition probably underlies the "power" of clairvoyants, but intuition is not magic; it is simply an enhanced ability of the brain to predict, based on past experience and limited current information.

I have done a lot of proofreading over the years, and somehow I have acquired the ability to recognize a typographical error in a page of print within a second of glancing at the page. I did not have this skill when I was younger. I have talked to other experienced editors who tell me that they also have developed this skill. I do not think that editors are naturally selected from people who have this talent. Rather, I believe that we can train our brains to scan in a way that far exceeds speed-reading. What fascinates me is that most typographical errors affect spelling, and I am a bad speller.


Neuroscientists are starting to learn where in the cerebral cortex different mental functions take place, but this knowledge has been a long time coming, and we still have far to go. However, some under-standing of the brain's activities has been available for a quite some time. For instance, ancient peoples knew that the brain controls move-ments of the body. The Edwin Smith Egyptian papyrus, dating to the seventeenth century BCE, describes a patient with paralysis of one side of the body (hemiplegia) resulting from a fractured skull. From the earliest time as well, it was recognized that injury to one side of the brain paralyzes the opposite side of the body. Today we know that one side of the cerebral cortex relates to the opposite side of the world, whether we are talking about movement, sensation, or vision.

In his 1664 book *Cerebri Anatome*, Thomas Willis (1621–1673), the great English physician and anatomist who is considered to be the father of neurology, describes the anatomy of the nervous system. (Incidentally, Sir Christopher Wren, the architect of London's St.

Paul's Cathedral, drew the illustrations for Willis's book.) Three years later, Willis initiated the study of neurological diseases in his book *Pathologicae cerebri, et nervosi generis specimen*. One of Willis's major contributions was the description of the blood vessels of the brain; his name is still remembered in the connection between the main arteries at the base of the brain, known as the Circle of Willis. As it turns out, diseases of the arteries of the brain underlie the most frequent brain illness: stroke.

Perhaps the most important discoveries in the field of neurology since the time of Willis have involved the "localization" of functions in the brain. We now know that different parts of the brain do different things. For example, perception of vision is localized to the area of the cerebral cortex at the back of the brain; the region that controls movement lies at the front of the brain.

The concept that different areas of the brain support different abilities began with the theory of phrenology, invented by Viennese anatomist and physician Franz Joseph Gall (1758–1828). Gall believed that specific talents, such as the ability to paint or to play music, could be read from bumps on the skull. This theory eventually was shown to be false—the outer shape of the skull does not represent what happens inside—but there is now strong evidence that different brain functions are localized in different areas of the cerebral cortex.

Paul Pierre Broca (1824–1880), a French physician and anatomist, discovered that words are organized into speech in the left frontal lobe of the brain. He studied the brain of a patient who had lost the ability to speak and found a stroke in the region that is now called Broca's area. Knowledge of the roles of individual areas of the brain originally came from postmortem examination of patients who had suffered strokes and other injuries that caused loss of a specific neurological function. Nowadays, we use magnetic resonance imaging (MRI) scans of the brain to investigate localization of an injury or disease.

Modern neurologists work in the opposite direction from Broca and others who discovered specific localization of different functions in the brain. Today's neurologists use the knowledge that those "giants" gave us to figure out where patients' symptoms are coming from. In this way, we deduce from a patient's symptoms where her stroke or tumor is situated. For instance, if the patient is unable to speak, there is probably damage to Broca's area in the left frontal lobe. If she is blind on the right side, then the left side of the visual system must be damaged.

## The left cerebral hemisphere: speech-language function

You will hear it said that the left cerebral hemisphere is "dominant." This means that the left hemisphere is the one where language abilities

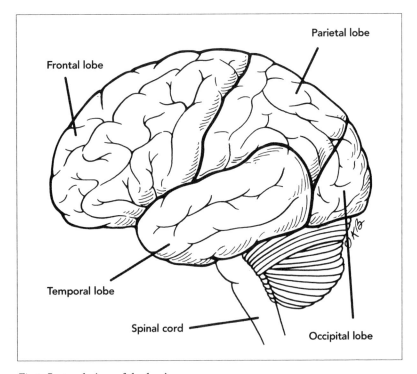

*Fig 1:* **Lateral view of the brain**

A lateral, or side, view of the brain shows the frontal lobe, responsible for conscious thought, the parietal lobe, involved in sensory perception, the temporal lobe, which processes smells and sounds, and the occipital lobe, which processes sight. The spinal cord transmits neural signals to and from the brain.

are located. Ninety percent of human beings are right-handed, and the language function of almost all right-handed people is located in the left cerebral cortex. Moreover, most of the 10 percent of the population who are left-handed use the left hemisphere for language.

Difficulty producing or understanding language is called dysphasia (sometimes aphasia). Someone with damage to Broca's area in the lower part of the left frontal cortex may understand everything that is said but have great difficulty speaking words or naming objects. He may be completely mute, or he may have very halting speech. This is called motor aphasia.

Broca's area is key to producing speech, but *understanding* speech takes place in Wernicke's area, further back in the left cerebral cortex at the junction of the parietal and temporal lobes. Damage to this area makes it difficult for a person to understand what is said and to follow spoken commands. This is called sensory or receptive aphasia. Although damage to Wernicke's area does not impair a person's ability to form words, it does prevent him understanding those words. Therefore most people with Wernicke's aphasia have fluent but incomprehensible garbled speech, sometimes called "word salad."

Reading is closely linked to speech. It is handled in the region between Wernicke's area and the left occipital visual cortex. Damage to this area may render a patient unable to read. This condition is termed alexia. (The term *dyslexia* is usually reserved for people who were born with developmental problems with reading.) Difficulty with writing, which is called dysgraphia, arises from damage between the reading area and the area in the left frontal lobe involved with hand movement.

The ability to do arithmetic is closely tied to reading. It is located somewhere near the reading center at the junction of the left parietal, temporal, and occipital lobes. In a later chapter, I will recount the story of a Greek bank manager whose first sign of brain cancer in this area was dyscalculia—the inability to calculate.

Despite what I have said about the localization of specific functions to particular areas of the brain, I must tell you that the information in the brain is distributed more widely than you might think. For instance, although visual information from the eyes travels mainly to the occipital cortex at the back of the brain, it also visits almost every other part of the cerebral cortex, where it helps to coordinate movement. Similarly, sensory fibers carrying impulses from the limbs and face go predominantly to the primary sensory cortex at the front of the parietal lobe, but these fibers also run to many other parts of the cerebral cortex, again to assist in the coordination of movement and many other mental processes.

Furthermore, the brain has an amazing plasticity. We see this when it heals after an injury. People who suffer a stroke or bullet wound to the brain in the left cerebral hemisphere may be completely unable to speak for weeks or months after the injury. However, most of the patients will partially recover as other parts of the brain take over the function of the part that was damaged.

## The frontal lobes: motor function

The frontal lobes of the brain, which lie behind the forehead, are the most recently developed parts of the human cerebral cortex in evolutionary terms. They contain many of our highest mental functions—those that are involved in social integration and the initiation of thought and action. Patients with damage to both frontal lobes are often disinhibited—prone to acting inappropriately in social situations. I have known patients with frontal lobe tumors or degenerations who shout for attention in a five-star restaurant, make passes at the wives of senior colleagues, and urinate in public. On the other hand, some patients with damage to the frontal lobes do not become disinhibited. Instead, they lose their motivation and become lethargic. Tumors, traumatic brain injuries, strokes, and brain degenerations may all cause frontal lobe syndromes.

The primary motor cortex is a strip of nervous tissue at the back of each frontal lobe. The strip runs from the bottom of the frontal lobe, up over the top of the brain, and down the middle part where it is adjacent to the opposite frontal lobe. The neurons of the primary motor cortex direct movement of the body—the motor cortex on the left side of the brain controls the right side of the body, and vice versa. Damage to one primary motor cortex paralyzes the opposite side of the body. Since movements of specific parts of the body are controlled by specific areas of the motor cortex, small lesions in different areas may have quite different effects. For instance, a stroke caused by blockage of one middle cerebral artery will paralyze the face and arm, but it will not affect the leg motor area because that region receives its blood supply from the anterior cerebral artery. On the other hand, a stroke due to blockage of the anterior cerebral artery will paralyze the opposite leg, but not affect the face and hand.

If a tumor or abscess irritates the motor cortex, a person may experience a focal epileptic seizure. The face and hand areas of the motor cortex are the largest—the neurological way of saying this is that they have the largest representation—because those parts of the body are capable of the most refined movements. Therefore, seizures arising from the motor cortex often begin in the opposite side of the face and hand.

To initiate a movement, the brain sends a message from the primary motor cortex in the posterior frontal lobe to the muscles of the opposite side of the body. However, the *decision* to make that move takes place somewhere else in the brain, perhaps in a region called the prefrontal cortex. This may be the location of free will or what we call the "mind." But it may also be that in the case of the brain, the whole is greater than the sum of the parts. Every part of the brain may be required to generate the mind.

Injury to the left parietal lobe may cause apraxia—the inability to make a movement or to copy it. Generally a neurologist tests for apraxia by asking the patient to show how he uses a toothbrush or to imitate the examiner using one. Apraxia may make it impossible for the patient to use his hand, even though the strength is intact. Apraxia is sometimes the most disabling feature of a stroke of the dominant cerebral hemisphere. A degenerative disease of the brain called corticobasal degeneration particularly affects motor memory of how to move the arm. As a result, the arm is apraxic and clumsy. Because this condition makes the patient feel that he does not know his own hand, the term *alien hand* has been given to this symptom.

When a person wants to make a rapid limb movement, such as reaching out and catching a ball, the nerve impulses responsible for that movement pass from the cerebral cortex down a group of specialized neurons called the corticospinal (or pyramidal) tract, located in the brain stem and spinal cord, to the motor neuron pools on the opposite side of the spinal cord. There the neurons translate the signals into movements of individual muscle groups.

Thus, a stroke affecting the primary motor cortex or corticospinal tract impairs the ability to make rapid movements of the opposite limbs and releases the reflexes in those limbs, so that they become greater than normal. A neurologist tests for reflexes by gently tapping a tendon, like the Achilles tendon at the ankle, and observing the resultant movement of the foot. If there has been damage to the corticospinal tract, then the reflexive movement is more dramatic than usual (the neurologist calls these "hyperactive reflexes"). The release of reflexes also makes the affected limbs stiff or spastic, which is why the patient has difficulty moving them rapidly.

On the other hand, when a person makes a slow, deliberate movement, the motor messages take an alternative route called the extrapyramidal pathways. These extrapyramidal messages go through a series of relay stations in the basal ganglia and cerebellum, where patterns of motor memories are stored and where the movement is refined. The motor patterns are integrated with sensory information returning from the body to the brain, and the result is the exquisitely elegant movement of a ballerina or the hand control of a portrait painter. Diseases such as Parkinson's disease, Huntington's disease, and cerebellar ataxia disrupt specific parts of the extrapyramidal system. Neurologists call this set of diseases the movement disorders.

*The parietal lobes: sensation*

The parietal lobes are fascinating parts of the brain. This is where we find the interpretation of sensation and the integration of complex artistic, spatial, and graphical functions. The parietal lobes—one on either side of the brain—are located behind the frontal lobes toward the top of the head above the ear.

The primary sensory cortex lies immediately behind and parallel to the primary motor cortex at the back of the frontal lobe. The primary sensory cortex receives sensory messages that tell the brain about touch, temperature, and pain on the opposite side of the body. Injury to the primary sensory area of the cerebral cortex results in loss of sensation on the opposite side of the body. Since the sensory cortex is arranged very much like the motor cortex, a small lesion of the sensory cortex results in loss of sensation in a specific part of the opposite side of the body. Thus, a stroke in the middle cerebral artery causes sensory loss in the opposite face and arm but does not affect sensation in the leg. As in the case of a motor stroke, the sensory abilities of the brain can recover after an injury. In fact, sensory abilities often recover more completely than the motor functions.

Just behind the primary sensory cortex is the sensory association area, which integrates the complex features of sensation. A patient with an injury to the hand sensory association area can feel touch or cold on the opposite hand normally, but he cannot recognize *where* that touch is located or *what* object is placed in the hand—for example, he cannot tell a dime from a quarter. Also, with his eyes closed he may be unable to recognize numbers drawn on the palm of the hand opposite the injury. (In a normal brain, this function is called graphesthesia.)

We often call people right-brained if they are sensitive, intuitive, and artistic, or left-brained if they are verbal, analytical, and likely to deal with the world logically. It is true that the interpretation of visual sensory input about spatial relationships is located primarily in the nondominant parietal lobe. In most people this area is on the right side, behind the sensory association area of the cerebral cortex. A patient with a stroke in this region may not be able to correctly locate cities on a map or to find her way in a familiar neighborhood because she has lost her geographical sense. Such a patient may be unable to draw or copy diagrams. Lesions in this area cause particular difficulty for people who rely on spatial skills, such as taxi drivers, artists, and architects. Because the location of visuospatial abilities is not as clearly one-sided as that of language, left-sided parietal lesions occasionally result in visuospatial problems.

The most disabling feature of a nondominant, usually right, hemisphere stroke is that the patient may have no awareness of the opposite, usually left, side of the world. This is called neglect. His eyes tend to look toward the right, and he fails to notice movements on the left. Even if tests reveal that his vision to the left side is intact, he continues to look to the right. A patient with neglect may leave his left arm hanging out of a jacket when getting dressed.

Lesions in the parietal and temporal lobes can seriously impair the highest level of interpretation of sensory inputs. These conditions are called agnosias, from the Greek *a-* meaning "not," *nosos* ("disease"), and *gnosis* ("knowledge"). For example, the patient may have lost the knowledge of what a toothbrush is or how it is used. This is very similar to the loss of motor memory that leads to apraxia.

One uncommon form of agnosia is prosopagnosia (from the Greek *prosopo*, meaning "face"). The patient is unable to recognize faces, even those of a parent, child, or famous film star. Patients describe the face as having a gray cloud across it. They can see the nose, the eyes, and the mouth, but the whole face is blurred and unrecognizable. Oliver Sacks describes such a patient in his book *The Man Who Mistook His Wife for a Hat*.

The lesion responsible for prosopagnosia is most commonly located in the inferior temporal lobe, usually on the right. Another problem associated with a right parietal lobe stroke is anosognosia, which literally means that the patient does not realize he has a problem. If I lift the paralyzed left arm of such a patient and ask him if there is anything wrong with it, he will recognize it as his own arm but deny that there is any problem.

*The temporal lobes: epilepsy and memory*

The temporal lobes—one on either side of the head—are responsible for the fascinating functions that underlie our most human capacities, such as memory, the senses of smell and hearing, imagination, hunger, sexual interest, and dreaming. The temporal lobes are situated just above the ears and deep to the temples. They lie below the frontal and parietal lobes, and in front of the occipital lobes at the back of the brain.

Patients with epileptic seizures that arise in the temporal lobes may experience various strange sensations and feelings, such as a prelude, or aura, to a seizure (I'll describe this in more detail in the chapter on epilepsy). Auras may include strange smells or tastes, snatches of music, weird feelings of familiarity (déjà vu) or confusion (jamais vu), or terrible fears. These sensations indicate that the temporal lobes play an important role in the interpretation of tastes, smells, and sounds. They also play a part in emotions and in the storage of memories.

When we remember a vivid event, we say that we can see it "in our mind's eye." Memory is perhaps the most complex function of the brain. We can recall events that happened fifty years ago, but no one knows where those memories are stored. One of Gary Larson's *Far Side* cartoons depicts a schoolboy asking his teacher if he can go home now because his brain is full. If you believe the message in this cartoon, you might think that we experience memory difficulties in later life because our brains are overfilled. This is not the case. Rather, Alzheimer's disease is caused by degeneration of the neurons, particularly those of the temporal lobes.

We store only a fraction of sensations coming into the brain. In his book *The Mind of a Mnemonist*, A. R. Luria (1902–1977), describes his studies of a patient named Solomon Shereshevskii, who had an extraordinary capacity for remembering things. Memories remained in Shereshevskii's brain much longer than normal, which made it difficult for him to concentrate on remembering new things. For Shereshevskii, the effort that he had to put into concentrating produced a mind that

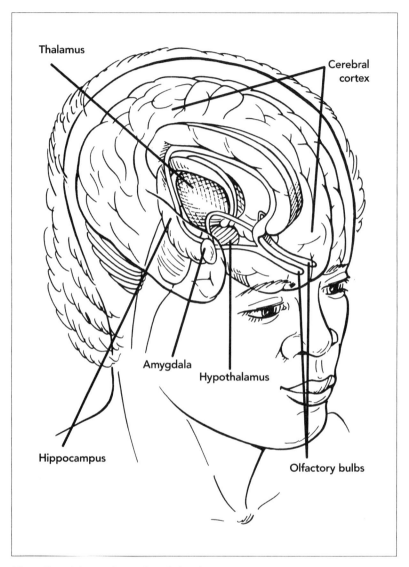

*Fig 2:* **Cognitive and emotional circuits**

Several important brain structures participate in thoughts and emotions: the hippocampus, involved in memory; the amygdala, in fear and aggression; the olfactory bulbs, processing smell; the hypothalamus, regulating heartbeat, respiration and other autonomic processes; the thalamus, relay station for sensory information coming into the brain, and the cortex, where input from all around the brain is assembled into thought.

was tormented and disorganized. We should be grateful that most memories fade quickly unless they are reinforced. Otherwise, we would all suffer from mental illness like Luria's patient.

Laying down new memories involves the formation of an engram, or memory trace, in the brain. The physical nature and location of this engram are unclear, however. Large parts of the brain can be damaged—by a stroke, for instance—without any one particular memory being lost. This must mean that there are multiple engrams of the same memory located in several places in the brain (this is sometimes called the principle of multiple redundancy). Exactly how the brain stores memories is unclear. The parts of the brain responsible for laying down new memories (the mammillary bodies, hippocampi, and forniceal systems) lie on the inner aspect of the temporal lobes and the upper brain stem. If both sides of this system are destroyed, the patient loses the ability to remember new facts. This condition is called Korsakoff's syndrome.

When I was a medical student, I saw a patient with Korsakoff's syndrome caused by severe alcoholism (the most common cause of the condition). When I asked him what he had for breakfast, he recited a list of items that seemed perfectly reasonable but turned out to be completely false. In providing me with this list, he apparently had pulled items from his memories of breakfasts past, before he had suffered the memory loss. His memories felt real, since he had no memory of this morning's breakfast to contradict his response.

Other brain injuries can produce Korsakoff's syndrome, including when a stroke is caused by blockage of the basilar artery, which is the main artery supplying both sides of the memory system at the back of the brain. One of the first patients to be treated for severe epilepsy by the neurosurgical removal of both medial temporal lobes was left with Korsakoff's syndrome.

Experts describe two main types of memories. Declarative memory is the ability to remember *who, what, and where*. Patients with Korsakoff's syndrome and Alzheimer's disease lose this type of memory. The declarative memory loss of Alzheimer's patients gets progressively worse with time. In Korsakoff's syndrome, however, the loss is usually permanent; it begins when the patient awakes from his last alcoholic binge. Patients with stroke may suffer memory loss, but usually they show some degree of recovery over time.

Procedural memory is motor memory, or the ability to remember *how*. This is the type of memory that a baby lays down when learning to walk. Motor memory underlies all learned motor skills, including those required to play sports. Motor memory loss occurs in patients with apraxia and causes walking difficulty in people with Parkinson's disease.

## The occipital lobes: vision

The main function of the occipital lobes—again, one on either side of the brain—is to enable a person to see what is going on around him. You may think that we use our eyes in order to see, but the eyes are really only the cameras through which we collect visual information. The primary visual cortex, at the very back of the occipital lobes, is where vision is actually perceived. What the eyes see is interpreted in the visual association areas in front of the primary visual cortex. This is where we find the neurons that detect the movement of a ball, for instance, and measure how fast it is traveling.

Even though the eyes are just the cameras serving the visual system of the brain, they are very complex structures. Eyes are exquisitely sensitive to certain electromagnetic waves, namely light waves from wavelengths of 400 (red) to 800 (violet) nanometers and they convert light energy into nerve impulses. The eye "sees" everything that sends it light from an arc of about 100 degrees in front of the face. Movement of the eyes extends this arc of vision to 180 degrees.

Because of the way that the eye and its lens are put together, light coming from the right half of the world strikes the left side of the retina of each eye. Nerve impulses that derive from the left half of the retina then travel along the optic nerve toward the brain. The nerve fibers carrying impulses from each left half of the two retinas come together to run side by side in the optic chiasm—the X-shaped junction of the two optic nerves—and then continue to the visual cortex of the brain's left occipital lobe. Therefore, the left visual cortex receives messages about light coming from the right half of a person's visual field. The opposite applies to light coming from the left.

A person who has an injury to one-half of the occipital cortex loses the perception of vision for the opposite side of the visual field. This is described as a hemianopia (or hemianopsia) and most commonly results from stroke, physical trauma, or a brain tumor. Because the lens of the eye turns light upside down, an injury to the upper part of one visual cortex results in loss of vision for the lower half of the opposite visual field (this is called a lower quadrantanopia). Many people with a hemianopia can learn to compensate for it.

The organization of vision in the occipital visual cortex is wonderfully elaborate. The center of the retina, called the fovea, has the highest density of color receptors called cones. Impulses from the fovea go to the rearmost part of the primary visual cortex, where the highest levels of visual acuity and color perception reside. When we look straight at letters or small objects, light is concentrated directly on the fovea. More peripheral parts of the retina have fewer cones and more black-and-white receptors, which are called rods. These peripheral areas, as well as the visual cortex to which they send impulses, have much lower visual acuity and poorer color perception. The peripheral areas function better in low-intensity light, which explains why it is easier to see a star if you look slightly to one side, rather than directly at it.

Because one eye is in a position slightly different from that of its twin, each eye receives a slightly different view of the world. This is the basis of stereoscopic vision, which is achieved by integration of the two eyes' nerve impulses when they reach the visual cortex and its adjacent visual association areas. If an object is far away, then the place where light from that object strikes the retina is essentially identical in both eyes. If the object is nearby, light from that object strikes the retinas in slightly different areas. Our brains use the integration and comparison of the impulses from each eye in order to see the world in 3-D and to judge distances.

Another important feature of the visual system is its ability to follow movement. The visual association areas determine an object's location in space at one moment in time and then again a few milliseconds later. This involves relatively simple physics, but it requires that the eye and brain be hardwired to connect the incoming signals from the retina with a series of movement-responsive neurons in the visual association areas. These neurons must do their work extremely rapidly. This is the basis of our being able to react to rapidly moving objects, such as when we catch a ball.

The physical separation of the movement-responsive neurons of the visual association areas from the location-responsive neurons of the primary visual cortex explains the problem of a fascinating patient I once worked with. She was blind as a result of degeneration of the primary visual cortex—she would walk straight into a wall—but she could still hit a moving tennis ball.

## The corpus callosum: alien hand syndrome

The cerebral cortex is divided into left and right halves. It is not the skull that holds the halves together; rather, it is a thick band of connective nerve fibers called the corpus callosum. Though the two cerebral cortices have many functions in common, other functions are unique to one or the other cortex. I have already pointed out that the right cerebral cortex specializes in artistic visuospatial activity, while the left deals particularly with speech and language. For the brain as a whole to work properly, each cerebral cortex must be able to talk to its partner. The brain achieves this communication through the corpus callosum. Damage to this structure may prevent this communication and produce what are called disconnection syndromes.

Research on patients with disconnection syndromes has taught us much of what we know about how the two sides of the brain interact. It also has provided insight into the "wiring diagram" of the brain. One patient's story will make this clear.

Clara, a sixty-year-old friend of mine, was helping her sick husband eat dinner in his hospital room. She had started to move the bed table toward him when she suddenly saw someone else's hand push the left side of the table. Shocked, Clara collapsed onto a chair. Then she received another fright. The strange hand followed her to the chair, folded itself into her lap and just lay there. Terrified, Clara used her right hand to touch this strange hand. Only then did she realize that the hand in her lap was her own left hand. After a few moments, the strange sense that it was someone else's hand disappeared.

Clara suspected that she was going mad. Later that evening, she called me to ask for advice. When I examined her the next day, I found absolutely nothing wrong with her nervous system. "Clara," I said, "You must have had an episode of what we call the alien hand syndrome."

"Well, it's bizarre you should call it that," she said, "because it was just like someone else, an alien, was there pushing the table and then putting her hand in my lap. What on earth caused it?"

I said, "To explain that, I need to tell you the story of a patient named Joe."

Joe was a gifted painter who had epilepsy. His seizures came three or four times a week. They would leave him unconscious for ten minutes. He would wet himself and become unable to paint for the remainder of the day. The seizures had severely affected Joe's schooling and social life.

No medication adequately controlled Joe's epilepsy. Eventually doctors investigated the possibility of surgery. Joe's epileptic discharges came from the left cerebral cortex near the speech area. The neurosurgeon concluded that he could not cut out this part of the brain for fear of taking away Joe's ability to speak. Instead, the neurosurgeon suggested an operation called a callosotomy, which involves cutting the corpus callosum. This prevents seizures from spreading from the left side of the brain to the right, thus reducing their severity.

Joe first experienced the alien hand syndrome three months after the callosotomy, when being tested in the office of his psychologist, Dr. Hyman. Joe had not had a grand mal attack for two months. He complained that his artistic talents had disappeared since the surgery, however. Dr. Hyman asked Joe to draw a picture, and it was clear that Joe was doing a poor job of it. Suddenly Joe's left hand reached over, grabbed the pencil from his right hand, and continued the drawing. Joe was astounded. He asked Dr. Hyman, "What in the world was that about? Whose hand was that?" Thinking quickly, Dr. Hyman said, "I think we have just seen an example of the alien hand syndrome."

Joe's artistic talents lay particularly in the right parietal lobe but he drew with his right hand. Therefore, until his surgery, the artistic centers in his right cerebral hemisphere had communicated through the corpus callosum to his left cerebral hemisphere the messages needed for the right hand to draw so beautifully. After the surgery cut the corpus callosum, those messages could no longer get through. The callostomy had separated Joe's artistic centers in the right hemisphere from the left hemisphere's control of his right hand. Disconnected from the artistic centers, Joe's right hand had become less creative.

When Joe's left hand slapped his right hand and grabbed the pencil, the left hand was expressing the frustration of the disconnected artistic right cerebral hemisphere at the aesthetic incompetence of the dominant left hemisphere. The right hemisphere could see the poor drawing— visual messages do not go through the corpus callosum, but instead go through pathways at the base of the brain. Due to the callosotomy, the right hemisphere could not send the messages to the left hemisphere to allow it to verbalize the problem. The right hemisphere could, however, make the left hand grab the pencil and take over the drawing.

Joe, thinking only with his verbal left hemisphere, knew that he had not sent any messages to move his left hand. In fact, the disconnected left hemisphere of his brain was only poorly aware of the left side of his body. When the left hand took away the pencil, it appeared to Joe as an alien's hand.

When I finished telling Clara about Joe, she at least understood that she was not going mad. However, I had to tell her that I did not know what had caused the disconnection in her case. It was obviously only temporary. Perhaps it was a migraine or a minor focal epileptic episode related to stress. Perhaps it was a tiny stroke (what we call a transient ischemic episode, or TIA), and the effects had cleared rapidly. Clara never had another attack of the alien hand syndrome.

*Connections between neurons in the cerebral cortex: synesthesia*

As the nervous system first forms in an embryo, it has many more neural connections than are present when the child is born. The excess connections are pared away, like the pruning of a tree, to allow the

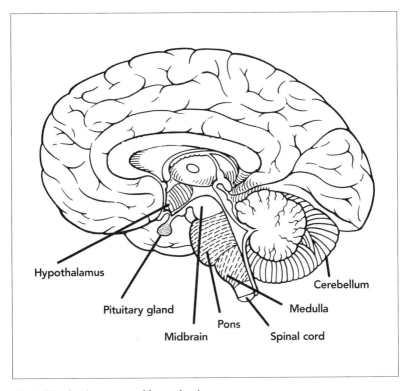

*Fig 3:* **The brain stem and lower brain**

In the brain stem, the pons and medulla regulate autonomic processes such as breathing, and, near the midbrain, the hypothalamus transmits internal and external signals to various parts of the brain and the pituitary gland releases hormones. The cerebellum helps coordinate movement and store movement memory.

individual parts of the brain to work independently and to carry out their specific tasks. Occasionally the pruning is incomplete, with bizarre results that would be totally unintelligible if we did not understand how the brain's cortical wiring developed. But a brilliant neuroscientist first shed light on this pruning process by figuring out a patient's weird condition. This condition is now called synesthesia—literally, "sensing things together."

Synesthesia is a rare disorder in which a person is born with an excessive spread of sensory information in the brain. The lack of "pruning" in brain development means that abnormal connections between neurons remain. As a result, one type of sensory stimulus not only stimulates the cortical sensory neurons that normally receive those messages, but also stimulates a second set of sensory neurons respon-sible for a totally different sensation. For example, synesthetes—people who have synesthesia—may hear a sound that instantly triggers an additional sensation, such as a color or a taste. Others may experience a sensation of touch associated with a particular visual pattern. Yet other synesthetes find that a particular musical note produces the additional perception of pain or a foul smell. Neurologist Richard Cytowic, who has written extensively about this condition, points out that there are many different types of synesthesia.

Children with synesthesia initially think that everyone perceives the world the way they do. They are puzzled when others view them as weird. Some children come to believe that they're mad, and they become secretive about their "strange" multiple sensations. When they learn there are others like them and read Cytowic's books, it is wonderful to see their relief.

One of my patients, Mrs. Brown, was born with synesthesia. She had abnormal connections between the neurons of the brain that normally recognize numbers and the neurons that normally recognize colors. Normally, a person looking at a number does not perceive an associated sensation of a color. But when Mrs. B looked at the number 3, it was green. She saw 5s as red, 8s as blue, and so on. Because of this, she could easily pick out the letter X spelled out in black 3s from a page covered in black 5s—she saw the 3s as green against a background of red 5s. For the rest of us, the same page would look like a mass of black 5s.

## Loss of sensory input into the brain: phantom limb sensations

People who have a leg or an arm amputated sometimes develop a sensation of severe pain in the missing limb. Some of these pain syndromes are caused by a neuroma—an overgrowth of regenerating nerve fibers coming from the cut stump of a nerve. The patient actually experiences pain in the missing limb, not in the stump. This is because the brain receives pain messages from the abnormally sensitive regenerated nerve fibers in the neuroma and interprets them as coming from the missing part of the limb, even though it has been amputated.

However, some patients without a neuroma have pains or other sensations that seem to come from the amputated limb. One patient may feel his amputated leg moving. Another may believe that her lost fingers are attached to the stump of her upper arm, and she can wiggle them. How does the brain produce these unusual sensations?

The research of V. S. Ramachandran, elegantly described in his book *Phantoms in the Brain*, indicates that these curious phenomena result from loss of sensory input to the brain. It appears that the brain "makes up" sensations to compensate for the lack of the normal sensory input. When people make things up, they are said to be confabulating, a term psychiatrists use to describe the replacement of fact with fantasy. It seems that the brain confabulates these strange phantom limb sensations. But, the brain is not "lying," and the patient is not voluntarily making up the pains or sensations.

The phenomenon of denervation supersensitivity explains what actually happens to amputees. Here is an example. If the nerves going to the bladder are destroyed, the bladder's smooth muscle cells become excessively sensitive to the chemical acetylcholine, which is normally released from the nerve endings to make the bladder contract. The smooth muscle cells, which are said to be denervated, increase the number of receptors for acetylcholine in an attempt to compensate for their lost nerves. This is what we call denervation supersensitivity. Similarly, the sensory neurons of the brain that previously received messages from an amputated limb develop denervation supersensitivity. They fire off in response to unrelated sensory inputs coming into the brain—or even in response to nothing at all. The firing of these sensory neurons leads the rest of the brain to believe that sensory impulses are coming from amputated body parts.

We do not know why some brains develop phantom sensations and others do not. I believe that this phenomenon is more common than we think. One of my patients, Mrs. Jones, was an eighty-year-old lady who complained that she was hearing music in her head. She had become increasingly deaf over the years, and I had to shout to get her to understand me. As she was talking, she suddenly broke off and said, "Excuse me a minute." She tilted her head to one side and smiled. After about twenty seconds she looked back at me and said, "I'm sorry. That was a piece from Handel's *Messiah*, and it was so lovely." I asked her if it was really the *Messiah*, or just something that sounded like music. She was adamant that she had heard a complete orchestra.

It is possible that Mrs. Jones was having epileptic seizures of an auditory type, but her electroencephalogram (EEG) and MRI brain scan were normal. It is also possible that Mrs. Jones was hallucinating due to a psychiatric illness, but she seemed perfectly sane to me. I thought she was experiencing one of the positive phenomena seen in patients with sensory deprivation. Mrs. Jones was becoming deaf, and her brain was making up for the loss of auditory input by pulling music from its memory bank.

Another of my patients had a much less pleasant experience resulting from the same phenomenon. She had suffered a mild head injury that damaged the olfactory nerve twigs at the top of the nose. She had lost her sense of smell. About three weeks after the injury, she began to perceive a constant, disgusting odor of rotting flesh. She saw several doctors, but they found nothing abnormal. The smell was not an epileptic aura; treatment with antiepileptic drugs did not help.

My patient eventually found a Web site for parosmia, the name given to this aberration of smell, and discovered that there are other sufferers in the world. One surgeon thought he could cure her condition by removing the olfactory mucosa at the top of her nose, but this did not help. I concluded that she was suffering from a phantom phenomenon in the brain. The sensory neurons for smell are located in an area called the piriform cortex. In my patient, these neurons had been cut off from their normal input of smell sensations and therefore were generating perceptions of bad odors. The only possible treatment was to remove the piriform cortex, but the patient decided against this major neurosurgical operation. I do not know if she followed my advice later; sometimes these phantom phenomena slowly disappear on their own.

Denervation supersensitivity probably underlies the strange visual phenomenon that I have experienced ever since I suffered a left retinal detachment. The operation to reattach my retina was successful, except that I was left with loss of the lower eighth of the visual field in my left eye. About six weeks after the surgery I was lying in bed, about to fall asleep. The room was dark. Suddenly I saw a white glow in the area where I had lost vision. This continues to happen whenever I am in the dark, particularly if I pay attention to it. The most striking thing is that when a door slams or some other unexpected noise startles me, the white area flares for a moment.

This curious phenomenon is another example of denervation supersensitivity. Neurons in my damaged left retina have become supersensitive. They fire off spontaneously, and the brain interprets this as a glow in the area of lost vision. The flare I experience with sudden noises is a bit like synesthesia. When an unexpected noise startles me, *every* neuron in my brain is stimulated, including the supersensitive neurons of the visual system. The sudden stimulation of my denervated visual neurons increases their discharge rate, thus producing the increased brightness of the glow.

# The Peripheral Nervous System

The peripheral nervous system consists of the nerves that run from the central nervous system—the brain and spinal cord—to the rest of the body. Two types of peripheral nerve fibers run to and from the spinal cord. Motor fibers run from the spinal cord to the muscles. Sensory fibers run from the skin, joints, and muscles to the spinal cord and brain stem.

There are two subsections of the peripheral nervous system: the autonomic nervous system and the cranial nerves. The autonomic nervous system comprises the nerves that run to and from the body parts that are outside our conscious control, such as the digestive system, heart, and blood vessels. Twelve pairs of cranial nerves serve everything above the neck—for example, the facial nerve carries motor fibers to move facial muscles, and the trigeminal nerve carries sensation from the face to the brain. (The first pair of cranial nerves, called the olfactory nerves, and the second pair, the optic nerves, are actually part of the central nervous system, though they are still called cranial nerves. The optic nerves carry messages from the eyes to the brain and the olfactory nerves carry nerve impulses related to smell.)

For most of their journey, peripheral nerves run in the limbs and trunk of the body. As they join the central nervous system, they run through the subarachnoid space, beneath the thick covering of the brain and spinal cord called the dura, where they are bathed in cerebrospinal fluid (CSF). The parts of the peripheral nerves within the dura are called the nerve roots. (Nerve roots may be compressed by a herniated intervertebral disc or a tumor. They may be damaged by chronic meningitis, in which pus is lying around them in the subarachnoid space.)

Peripheral nerves are like electric cables. The wires are the axons. Some axons have a fatty covering called the myelin sheath. These are called myelinated nerve fibers. The myelin sheath spiraling around the axon is actually part of a supporting cell called the Schwann cell. The

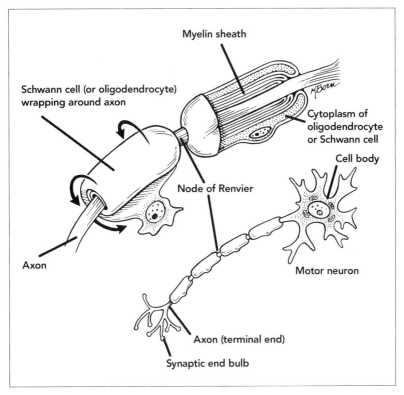

*Fig 4:* **Motor neuron and myelin**

The motor neuron carries the brain's signals for the body to move. The myelin sheath on a neuron's axon, like insulation on an electrical wire, helps speed the signal along the axon.

myelin sheath insulates the electrical impulse traveling along the axon. This helps myelinated nerve fibers conduct nerve impulses rapidly (10 to 60 meters per second depending upon the fiber's diameter). Large-diameter myelinated fibers include motor fibers, which go to the skeletal muscles, and sensory fibers, which carry information about touch, joint position sense, and vibration sense toward the spinal cord. Myelinated fibers with smaller diameters convey sensations of sharp pain.

Axons that have no myelin sheath are termed nonmyelinated or unmyelinated nerve fibers. These fibers conduct nerve impulses slowly, at less than one meter per second. There are two types of nonmyelinated fibers in the peripheral nervous system. Sensory fibers carry nerve impulses for pain toward the central nervous system. Autonomic fibers carry nerve impulses to control the gut or the blood vessels.

The peripheral nerve fibers are extraordinary. The longest motor fibers run from the motor neuron at the lower end of the spinal cord to the foot muscles. These axons are about 36 inches long in an adult man. The cell body that the axon is part of is less than 0.2 millimeters in diameter. If you were to magnify this cell body to the size of a man's head, the man's body would be more than one mile tall and about four millimeters in diameter.

Two kinds of unmyelinated fibers can be up to 36 inches long, but their diameter is one-twentieth the size of the large myelinated nerve fibers. Some of these tiny fibers carry messages from the neurons beside the spinal cord in the small of the back (the lumbar region) to the blood vessels of the feet. Others carry burning pain and temperature sensation from the feet to the spinal cord It is amazing that such delicate structures can hold together, let alone tell the brain when the foot has stepped on a hot coal.

The extraordinary length of the peripheral nerve fibers imposes a tremendous burden on the neurons and axons. All the proteins that make up the nerve fiber are produced in the neuron cell body, and they have to be exported all the way down the axon to its end. A process called axonal transport moves these proteins, as well as tiny cell parts called mitochondria (mitochondria make the high-energy compounds essential for the life of all cells).

The transport mechanisms require energy produced by the mitochondria, as well as the participation of many different "molecular motors." These motors act like railway engines linked to boxcars that carry the "freight"—proteins and submicroscopic organelles like mitochondria. The "trains" move along microtubules, which act like railway lines in the axon. The trains all move at different speeds, some in one direction and some in the other.

The axonal transport system in the peripheral nerves works at maximum capacity because of the thinness of the axons and the distances involved. If disease impairs the supply of proteins to the nerve fiber endings, the nerve endings wither away. At the ends of the very longest fibers, the result will be loss of sensation and motor function in the hands and feet. This explains why patients with most diseases of the peripheral nerves complain of numbness and weakness that starts in their toes and fingers. The technical term for this is length-dependent axonal polyneuropathy, or dying-back neuropathy. This is just one type of peripheral neuropathy that may be caused by many different diseases that I will discuss in chapter 12.

The Schwann cells that form the myelin sheaths are also at the limits of their metabolic capacity. Thousands of Schwann cells lie along the axon. Each makes a segment of the sheath, from the beginning of the axon to its ending. If disease compromises Schwann cell metabolism, the myelin breaks down. Depending on the role of the nerve cell that has been demyelinated, the results range from pain to paralysis.

## The Brain and Sports

In this chapter I have described how the nervous system is intricately organized to give us an extraordinary range of abilities. In large part, however, I have focused on how these abilities may be impaired in patients with neurological diseases. Before I leave this chapter I would like to show you how all these parts of the nervous system accomplish some of the unique feats that humans are capable of. To me, some of the finest examples occur in top athletes. Most of us indulge in sports at some level. Some time ago, my own less-than-Olympian abilities got me thinking about how the brains of top athletes help produce their almost superhuman performances.

Top male tennis professionals can serve the ball at more than 150 miles per hour. This is an incredible feat of neurological coordination. One hand throws the ball up, while the racquet in the other hand circles back and comes over to hit the ball just as it starts to fall from the zenith of the throw. The toss of the ball and the swing of the racket have to be coordinated with the movements of the head and eyes to monitor the track of the ball, and with the movements of the body and legs to swing the player's weight behind the serve. At the top of the swing, the server must hit the ball in a spatial window that is no more than four square inches in size, and he must do so in a time window of less than a millisecond. Less than one second goes by between the server's decision to throw the ball and the moment he hits it.

Let us look at the neurological processes that allow top-flight tennis players to hit a 150-mph ace. The neuronal pathways that carry messages in the nervous system are not like electric wires running from one end of the nervous system to the other. Rather, the messages travel through a series of individual nerve cells separated by gaps called synapses. The maximum speed of conduction of an impulse by a human nerve fiber is about 60 meters per second, which interestingly is nearly the speed of the fastest tennis serve. At a synapse, the nerve impulse is carried from one neuron to the next by the release of a puff of a chemical called a neurotransmitter. The nerve impulse takes a few milliseconds to pass across a synapse.

The message to start a tennis serve travels from that part of the brain we call the "volitional center," where our decisions are made, to the motor cortex and down the spinal cord to the muscles of the arms and legs—a distance of up to two meters. If the message were to pass from the brain's volitional center directly to the muscles of the legs, traversing three or four neurons and their synapses, it would take about 40 milliseconds for the muscles to contract. However, this direct communication would simply produce a twitch of the leg muscles, rather than the finely controlled body movements that result in a 150-mph serve.

Instead, the brain performs a whole series of tasks to start the serve. The nervous activity underlying even a simple movement is much more complex than the activity that generates a simple twitch. First, the brain generates an electrical potential called the readiness potential, which can be detected in an electroencephalogram 500 to 1,000 milliseconds before the movement is initiated. Conscious awareness of the decision to make a movement occurs about 300 milliseconds before the actual movement begins. The nerve impulses travel from the motor cortex to a series of motor control centers, including the basal ganglia near the center of the brain, the cerebellum at the back of the brain, and the motor centers of the spinal cord. Each of these motor control centers "talks" to several other control centers. The brain says, "Do it!" and the motor control centers translate the message into smooth, integrated movements of many muscles and joints. The server hits the tennis ball.

Also important in fine-tuning the server's movements are the feed-back systems from the muscles and joints, as well as the balance mechanisms related to the inner ear and the eyes that provide the brain with real-time information. I do not know how many neurons are involved in this whole process, but 50 is a good guess. The total transit time for the nerve impulses traveling through these 50 neurons and their synapses may be 500 milliseconds. This is about the length of time that the server has available to achieve the whole coordinated movement of the serve.

Now let us think about the brave receiver on the other side of the net. He has only about a half a second between the moment when the server hits the ball and the moment when he must have his racket in exactly the right place, traveling with the correct speed and held at the perfect angle to return the ball out of the reach of the advancing server. The receiver needs to know, in the shortest time possible, where the ball is going to bounce on his side of the court. This means that the receiver's brain must calculate the trajectory of the ball in less than 100 milliseconds, leaving him 400 milliseconds to initiate and complete the coordinated movements needed to return the ball. He has to determine where the approaching ball will bounce to within three inches if he is going to be in position to hit it back. This three-inch margin of error requires the receiver to read the serve to an accuracy of about 10 minutes of angle (one minute is one-sixtieth of a degree of angle) in the first foot or two of the ball's flight.

The serve receiver's visual system tracks the ball as nerve impulses from the image of the ball on the retina pass to a relay station at the base of the brain, called the lateral geniculate body, and then to the visual association areas of the brain's occipital lobe. There, movement-sensing neurons calculate the direction and speed of the tennis ball by correlating several "pictures in time" of the ball. Then the neurons send the information to the motor control centers to initiate the body movements necessary to return the serve. Since at least five neurons and synapses lie between the retinal cones and the motor activation center of the serve receiver, and since each visual image takes about 25 milliseconds to reach the neurons interpreting the angle of the serve, his brain can collect very few pictures in the 100 milliseconds he has before it's time to return the ball. Pity the poor receiver; it is little wonder that a 150-mph serve is often an ace.

In baseball, the odds are even more stacked against the nervous system. A batter faces the task of using a round bat to hit a ball traveling at 90 mph. A pitcher's fastball reaches home plate in less than half a second. The batter has to use the same visual and neurophysiological processes as the tennis receiver to estimate where the ball will go before he initiates his swing.

A baseball is less than 2.9 inches in diameter, and a bat's maximum diameter is 2.75 inches. Both the ball and the bat are circular in cross section. In order to hit a home run, the batter must achieve contact with the two diameters exactly in line. If the swing is half an inch too low, it results in a fly ball. Half an inch too high, and he hits a ground ball. If the batter swings five milliseconds too early, then the ball goes foul toward third base. Five milliseconds too late, and he fouls towards first base. The batter's "sweet zone" for a home run is less than an inch in height and three inches from the end of the bat, which itself is located three feet from his hands. The ball spends only 10 milliseconds within that zone. (I should note that the "sweet zone" has nothing to do with the regulation strike zone, which is about three feet high and seventeen inches wide.) Given the challenges that batters face, it is astounding that some can achieve 260 hits and 70 home runs in a season.

In order to catch a fly ball traveling at 50 to 100 mph, a fielder must solve a four-dimensional problem to move himself—and his glove—to a six-square-inch area many yards from where he started. The brain of the fielder must make a series of four-dimensional calculations based upon visual information coming from his eyes. Then the brain must process these calculations in the same way as the tennis receiver. The baseball fielder has four or five seconds to make these calculations, as he simultaneously runs and alters his direction in relation to the angular movement of the baseball.

I ask you, what separates an amateur from a professional athlete? Innate ability and practice. Innate ability must come from the athlete's particular combination of genes that relate to speed of conduction of nerve impulses along nerves and to the complexity of the motor control centers. Practice and memory also play an important part in helping the athlete reach the pinnacle of performance. The memory of a movement is called the motor engram. Many motor engrams are located in the cerebral cortex, basal ganglia, cerebellum, and spinal cord. The more often we make movements, the more firmly laid down are the motor engrams. However, most engrams fade slowly and need to be reinforced constantly if they are to remain. This is the neurological basis of the aphorism "practice makes perfect." And it helps athletes stay at the top of their game.

## Chapter 2

# Alzheimer's Disease

One day, two patients came to see me with complaints of memory problems. They turned out to have very different conditions.

Señor Alonzo (not his real name) had come all the way from Argentina to see me because he could not get a clear answer about his problem from neurologists in his own country. He was a seventy-one-year-old businessman who ran several successful companies in Buenos Aires. Sr. Alonzo complained that his memory was deteriorating and he feared he was developing Alzheimer's disease. I joked with him that we neurologists have an aphorism: "If the patient comes complaining about his memory, the diagnosis is not Alzheimer's disease." And that proved to be true in Sr. Alonzo's case. He told his story very clearly, in excellent English, and was able to tell me everything about his businesses and his social life.

"I am having real trouble remembering the names of business acquaintances and family friends when I meet them," he told me. "I know their faces, but I just can't get their names! I have never been very good at names, but it is getting much worse lately. Also, I keep finding that I am having difficulty finding words. All this is very embarrassing."

I put Sr. Alonzo through a battery of mental tests and thoroughly examined his nervous system. All was normal. He remembered three objects—a bicycle, a pencil, and a rose—three minutes after I had occupied him with other mental tasks. I also tested his ability to repeat single-digit numbers forward and backward—a good test for mental function. Innately intelligent and mathematically inclined people can repeat more numbers forward than those who are less bright. On the other hand, the ability to turn the numbers around and repeat them backward is a better test of the memory. Sr. Alonzo correctly repeated eight digits forward and six digits backward.

I said, "Señor, your memory and mind are better than mine! I *also* have some trouble finding people's names and the right word sometimes. And I am younger than you."

"Ah, yes," he replied, "but you don't realize that my mind was so sharp when I was younger, and it is just not the same now."

I told Sr. Alonzo a little story that I have found useful in explaining normal aging of the brain. In the game of memory, fifty-two playing cards are spread out facedown, and players turn over any two cards to see if they can make a pair. If the player does not make a pair, the cards are turned facedown again and the next player takes a turn. When a player turns up a particular card—let's say it's an ace—and remembers that another ace was turned over earlier, the player only needs to remember the location of the second ace in order to make the pair. Simple? Yes. But a twelve-year-old will beat an adult in a game of memory, and an eight-year-old will beat a teenager. At young ages, the brain is especially designed to recognize and remember patterns.

Now contrast the game of memory with the case of elderly wise men in China. The Chinese revere their elders and respect their elders' wisdom. In ancient times politicians would present complex problems of diplomacy to the elders. Such problems are like a game of chess, with many possible ways to approach them and many potential solutions. The elders would ponder the problem for a while and then pronounce a course of action that the politicians would follow—usually with success. The key point is that the Chinese elders sometimes had such poor memories that they would forget the problem an hour later.

Our brains continually change throughout our lifetime. As newborn babies, we have 100 billion ($10^{11}$) neurons in our brains. We lose about 85,000 neurons a day from birth onward, mainly due to simple aging. However, our minds do not go completely downhill after birth. In fact, our brains get better with age, at least for a time, or else we would not use phases like "growing up" and "becoming an adult." The synapses that I described in the previous chapter continue to be created and changed during our lifetime. This may provide one of the mechanisms for laying down memories.

After I told my story to Sr. Alonzo, I looked him in the eye and said, "Your brain is not the same as it was when you were twenty, and you should be grateful. You may not have such a good memory, but your knowledge and judgment are much better. Your memory is considerably better than most seventy-one-year-olds. You do not have Alzheimer's disease." Sr. Alonzo went back to Argentina only partly convinced, and I continued to see him once a year to reassure him. Ten years later, he was still in charge of several companies, though he had handed over much of the day-to-day management to his sons. He had not developed progressive Alzheimer's disease.

Mrs. Abramowitz was the other patient that day. She sat at my desk as her daughter, Betty, talked to me. Mrs. Abramowitz seemed disengaged; she gazed around the office and looked out the window. Betty said that she was worried about her mother's memory. Last week her mother had lost her way when driving to Betty's house, a journey she had made hundreds of times. Mrs. Abramowitz would ask how the children were and then ask the same question again five minutes later. She had lost her purse several times and was regularly forgetting to lock up her house when she went out.

Like Sr. Alonzo, Mrs. Abramowitz was seventy-one. When I tested her memory she remembered only one out of three objects after three minutes, and that only with prompting. She tried to explain this away: "I don't need to pay attention to silly games like that." She repeated six digits forward but only three backward, suggesting that she was bright but had problems laying down new memories. When I asked her why she was seeing me today, she replied, "I thought we were going to the mall!"

Sadly, Mrs. Abramowitz's clinical diagnosis was Alzheimer's disease. When we look at the brains of people like Mrs. Abramowitz after they die, more than three-quarters of the brains will have the changes of Alzheimer's disease. Half of those brains will also have signs of little strokes. Most likely, both these conditions contributed to the patients' memory problems.

When I had finished examining Mrs. Abramowitz, I said to Betty, "Sadly, I have to confirm your suspicions," though we had not yet used the term *Alzheimer's disease*. I turned to Mrs. Abramowitz and said, "Unfortunately, you do have some problems with your memory." She did not seem very interested in the information. I took her out into the waiting room, where my secretary could keep an eye on her while I talked to Betty.

## Clinical Features of Alzheimer's Disease

Alzheimer's disease is characteristically a disease of the elderly, so much so that it used to be called senile dementia. It once was considered different from a similar disorder, presenile dementia, which occurs in people under sixty years of age. We now know that these are the same disease, though for younger-onset cases the condition is more likely to be familial (that is, others in the family had the same disease, often one parent, a grandparent, and perhaps a sibling) and to have a genetic basis. Alzheimer's disease is also common in patients with Down's syndrome (mongolism). In their case, it can occur as young as thirty years of age.

Alzheimer's is a slowly progressive disorder. It is often initially indistinguishable from the normal, age-related decline of memory mentioned earlier. Gradually, however, the memory lapses become more frequent and obvious to people who spend time with the patient. The patient himself often is less aware of the memory lapses and makes excuses to explain them: "Oh! I didn't hear you. Maybe my deafness is getting worse." Patients are often very good at covering up their symptoms, particularly if they are intelligent. I helped look after an eminent bishop who was totally unaware of the date, as well as the fact that he was in a hospital. Whenever I visited him in his hospital room he would say, with charming grace, that he would call his housekeeper to get tea for us. He was seemingly unconcerned that he was wearing a hospital gown. When I asked him why he was dressed this way, he replied, "Oh! I got up late this morning."

Initially Alzheimer's disease does not affect the cognitive capacities. A patient may have good judgment and ability to reason but has deterioration of memory. Her capacity for naming begins to fail, first for names of people but later for everyday objects. Geographical capacity is often the next to falter; like Mrs. Abramowitz, the patient may get lost driving to a familiar location or forget her car's location in a parking lot. Soon the patient begins repeatedly asking loved ones the same question and denying that the question was answered only a few minutes earlier. Accidents begin to happen; the patient may leave food to burn on the stove or find herself locked out of the house because she forgot her keys. Patients with Alzheimer's disease are prone to motor vehicle accidents and must eventually be persuaded to stop driving.

Alzheimer's disease most commonly presents symptoms like those of Mrs. Abramowitz, but it can paint a number of different clinical pictures. Another common presentation is confusion in an elderly person who goes into the hospital for an unrelated event.

Morris, a friend of mine from Boston, called me about his seventy-five-year-old stepfather, Alvin, who was in just this situation. Alvin was in a hospital with pneumonia. The doctor had told the family that Alvin had advanced Alzheimer's disease, that his wife should sign a DNR (do not resuscitate) order, and that they should stop all the antibiotics and let him die peacefully. Morris, who is an eminent attorney, said, "But Alvin can't have advanced Alzheimer's disease. It does not come on that quickly. We saw him just a few weeks ago, and he was joking around, as sharp as a tack. His memory might not be as good as it used to be, but he was certainly not demented at that time."

At Morris's request I spoke to Alvin's neurologist, a competent doctor, who said it was clear that Alvin was demented. He was thrashing around in his hospital bed and it was impossible to prevent him injuring himself without physical restraints and a lot of drugs. I was sure that the diagnosis of Alzheimer's disease was premature. The only hope was for me to transfer Alvin to my hospital in Miami, withdraw all drugs, and have his wife and a nurse stay with him twenty-four hours a day till his elderly brain got over the effects of the infection, being deprived of sleep in the hospital setting, and the many drugs he had been given that had confused his mind. I told the staff that it would be a very difficult four days, and it was. However, at the end of that time, Alvin became lucid, got over his pneumonia and other metabolic problems, and went home.

Every year for the next five years, at Alvin's birthday party his family would toast me as "the god who gave Alvin back to them." Over the years I have had a dozen patients whom I have "brought back from the dead" like this, simply by recognizing that the elderly brain does not do well in the hospital. Infections, anemia, changes in blood chemistry, medications, and sleep deprivation can add up to cause what is sometimes called ICU- (intensive care unit) or hospital-induced psychosis. Though such a reaction can occur in young people, it is most common in the elderly. Of those who experience this type of temporary dementia (better termed an acute confusional state), most do have age-related deterioration of the brain that may eventually lead to Alzheimer's disease, and the ICU psychosis has uncovered the disease several years before it otherwise would have been discovered.

The best thing for a patient like Alvin is to stop as many medications as possible and to have a family member with the patient all the time.

Patients who have not recovered completely from whatever brought them into hospital should nevertheless be discharged to the familiar surroundings of home as soon as possible.

Most patients with Alzheimer's disease begin with memory problems and progress to loss of other higher intellectual functions, such as judgment. However, in a few patients the initial symptom might be a more isolated problem, such as a specific loss of language ability. Alan was just such a patient. He was a fifty-eight-year-old Vermont attorney who came to see me with his thirty-four-year-old wife, Margaret. They showed me pictures of their two young daughters, ages two and three. I immediately knew that something was wrong because, although Alan pulled out the pictures and gesticulated vigorously during our conversation, it was Margaret who did all the talking. In fact, Alan said not a word because he had lost the ability to talk.

About six months earlier, Alan had begun having difficulty finding the right word when speaking. This is a major problem for an attorney. Gradually his speech had become more halting and telegraphic, though he understood everything that was said to him. Eventually he completely lost the power of producing speech. By the time I first saw him, he was having considerable difficulty with writing, though his abilities to read and to understand verbal communications remained intact.

Having realized that something serious was happening to him, Alan came to see me because he was preparing a new will. Margaret was his second wife, and the divorce from his first wife had been bitter. Alan wished to leave everything to his new wife and daughters when he died, but he predicted that his first wife would contest the new will because of his inability to speak or write.

This problem intrigued me. I knew from the records of other doctors who had investigated Alan that a stroke or tumor had been ruled out. He seemed to be suffering from a progressive degenerative brain disease with atrophy of the language area on the left side of the brain. We call this a focal atrophy of the brain.

I was able to prove through testing—despite the difficulties of doing so without the benefit of spoken language—that Alan's cognitive and memory functions were preserved. He understood complex commands and was able to communicate surprisingly well with gestures. In this way he confirmed that he wanted to leave nothing to his first wife and that he knew exactly what his estate was worth. He was clearly competent and capable of formulating his desires, taking actions to achieve these desires, and understanding the implications of those actions. I made copious notes and provided him with a letter summarizing my findings and my conclusion that he was competent to make a will.

Today we call Alan's problem primary progressive aphasia (loss of language function), but at the time I first saw him the condition had not been well described. We now know that primary progressive aphasia can be caused by several different progressive neurological degenerations, Alzheimer's disease being the most common.

A couple of years later, I moved to the University of Miami and lost contact with Alan. Five years later, I received a letter from his attorney saying that Alan had died recently, having developed a progressive dementia that started a year after I saw him. The letter asked me to provide an affidavit that when I had seen him originally, he was competent to make a will. As Alan had anticipated, his will was being contested. I wrote the affidavit, and the petition from his former wife to throw out the new will was rejected by the probate court.


Violet was another patient who, like Alan, probably had the focal atrophy version of Alzheimer's disease. In her case, however, the atrophy started at the back of the brain, in the visual cortex. Violet was in her sixties and had been a semiprofessional tennis player. A year earlier she had begun to complain of blurred vision, which gradually had progressed to blindness. The ophthalmologist had found nothing wrong with her eyes and had referred her to a community neurologist. The neurologist had suggested that Violet's problem was hysterical blindness because she could see his hand moving in front of her face.

As I teach doctors in training, you diagnose hysteria at your peril, particularly in the elderly.

Violet's daughters gave me an extraordinary addition to her story. Violet insisted that she could not see anything, but when they took her to the tennis court and threw a ball to her, she could hit it. This seemed unlikely to me because I had just seen her walk into the wall as she was being led to my office door. To check the daughters' story, I threw Violet a ball of paper. To my amazement, she caught it.

After a good deal of additional testing, I came to the conclusion that Violet's blindness was caused by degeneration of her primary visual cortex, the posterior part of the brain that receives nerve impulses coming from the eyes and translates them into the perception of vision. On the other hand, it seemed likely that the visual association area—the area of the brain, just in front of the primary visual cortex, where the neurons that interpret movement are found—must have remained intact. This allowed her brain to perceive the moving tennis ball, even though she could not visually perceive objects that were not moving.

Over the next year Violet gradually lost the ability to "see" even moving objects. She then progressively lost her memory and her ability to speak. It was clear that the degeneration was spreading slowly forward in the brain. She later started having attacks that contorted her face and body as though she was in terrible pain. She died about five years after the first visual symptom.

## What Is Alzheimer's Disease?

Alzheimer's disease is an epidemic in developed countries, where people are living longer, because it becomes increasingly common as a population ages. Nearly 50 percent of people who reach the age of eighty-five will have symptoms of Alzheimer's dementia. At least five million people in the United States currently have dementia, and the number may increase to 13 million by 2050. Almost half the patients in American nursing homes have dementia. Alzheimer's disease costs Medicare nearly $100 billion a year. In addition to the cost to the health care system, the disease imposes an enormous burden on the patients' families.

Senile dementia is not a new disease. Edward III of England (1312–1377) is believed to have died of this condition. Shakespeare describes dementia well in his play *As You Like It*:

All the world's a stage,
And all the men and women merely players …
Last scene of all,
That ends this strange eventful history,
Is second childishness and mere oblivion,
Sans teeth, sans eyes, sans taste, sans everything.

Eighteenth-century physicians found softening of the brain, presumably the result of strokes, in people who had died after suffering dementia. Then, in 1906, Alois Alzheimer (1864–1915) described a fifty-one-year-old woman who experienced memory loss, paranoid delusions, and progressive aphasia (the inability to form words). Alzheimer examined the patient and then performed an autopsy to study her brain after she died. The outer aspect of her brain, the cerebral cortex, had shrunk. When he applied silver stains to sections of her brain—a new technique in Alzheimer's day—he found the changes that we now consider diagnostic of the disease named after him: neurofibrillary tangles and plaques.

Neurofibrillary tangles and plaques are masses of insoluble protein deposited in and around neurons of the cerebral cortex. We say that these masses are precipitated because it is as though they have crystallized out of solution. The protein masses in neurons are called neurofibrillary tangles, and the masses in the tissue outside the neurons are called neuritic or senile plaques.

Several different proteins make up plaques and tangles, but our current thinking is that one of them, beta-amyloid, is the main culprit. Beta-amyloid is formed from a larger protein, amyloid precursor protein. When beta-amyloid is deposited in the brain it damages the neurons, first by destroying the synapses and the fine branches of neurons called dendrites. The loss of dendrites and synapses reduces the brain's ability to do the millions of computations per second that underlie normal intellectual function. Eventually, the precipitated proteins kill many of the neurons. Since the process of precipitation of beta-amyloid usually starts in the hippocampus—the part of the brain involved in storing new memories—loss of short-term memory is the earliest sign of Alzheimer's disease.

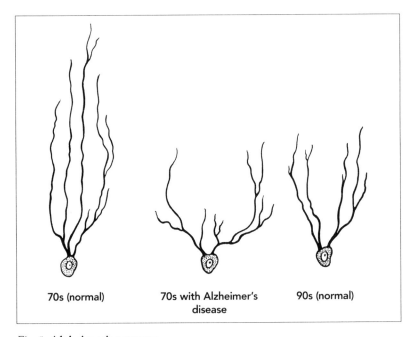

| 70s (normal) | 70s with Alzheimer's disease | 90s (normal) |

*Fig. 5:* **Alzheimer's neurons**

This diagram compares the neurons and their dendrites of a healthy 70-year-old person, a 70-year-old patient with Alzheimer's disease and a healthy 90-year-old person. In Alzheimer's disease, the neurons lose more dendrites than would be lost by a normal person 20 years older.

Here is the $64,000 question: What causes the production of beta-amyloid from amyloid precursor protein? Is it "normal aging?" (This would not tell us much, since we understand little about normal aging.) Is it some environmental factor that most of us are exposed to, such as insecticides or air pollution? Twenty years ago a popular theory was that Alzheimer's disease was caused by aluminum, because injections of aluminum salts into the brains of rabbits produced neurofibrillary tangles similar to those associated with Alzheimer's disease. When I was giving talks to Alzheimer's disease support groups at that time, I was always asked about this theory. Since I was not convinced that the theory was true (and later research confirmed it was not), I would answer, "Well, I am still cooking with aluminum pots!"

Some rare families suffer from an inherited form of Alzheimer's disease. These patients begin to experience symptoms in their forties— much earlier than in most nonfamilial cases. Research scientists called neurogeneticists have shown that some members of these families have mutations of the gene for amyloid precursor protein. Other family members have mutations of genes for other proteins, such as the secretases and presenilin, which are enzymes involved in the brain's process for disposing of amyloid precursor protein.

The gene apolipoprotein E predisposes people to developing Alzheimer's disease. Someone who bears two copies of a certain form of this gene, ApoE4, has a substantially increased risk of developing Alzheimer's disease in later life compared with people who have one of the other two forms, ApoE3 and ApoE2.

Amyloid precursor protein is normally located at the membrane of the neuron. Its job is still unclear, but normally, when this protein's work is done, enzymes break it up and dispose of it without producing brain damage. If the protein itself has an abnormal structure, as in families with a mutation of its gene—or, to a lesser extent, as a person ages—the disposal process becomes abnormal. This leads to the precipitation of beta-amyloid.

The brains of normal elderly people contain some plaques and tangles of beta-amyloid, but far fewer than those with established Alzheimer's disease. Perhaps this explains why all our memories worsen as we get older, and why we suffer "senior moments"—a person's name is on the tip of our tongue, but we just cannot bring it to the forefront of our conscious mind. Strangely, the memory often resurfaces later, when we are not even searching for it. The person's name was not lost; it was just hiding, though we do not know where! The problem of "senior moments" is called benign senile forgetfulness or an age-related memory problem.

Minimal cognitive impairment (MCI) is a condition that lies between benign senile forgetfulness and true Alzheimer's disease, in terms of both the patient's mental problems and the amount of neuro-fibrillary degeneration and plaque formation in the brain. In the case of Mrs. Abramowitz, her mental lapses were clearly symptoms of Alzheimer's disease.

## Tests for the Diagnosis of Alzheimer's Disease

After I led Mrs. Abramowitz into the waiting room, her daughter Betty stayed with me in the consultation room. I told her much of what I have just told you about Alzheimer's disease. She responded, "How can we be sure, doctor?"

I told Betty that best way to be sure is through neuropsychological testing, which can show exactly which brain functions are impaired and how badly. Alzheimer's disease generally causes a characteristic pattern of impairment of mental performance on these tests.

There is currently no reliable blood test for Alzheimer's disease. A brain biopsy definitively confirms the diagnosis, but it is very invasive to drill a hole in the skull and remove a piece of brain to study under the microscope. This procedure seems especially undesirable when there is no effective treatment. In rare cases brain biopsy can reveal a treatable cause of dementia—for example, inflammation of the blood vessels—but there was very little likelihood of one of those conditions in Mrs. Abramowitz's case.

I told Betty that I would arrange some less invasive tests—including blood studies for thyroid function, vitamin $B_{12}$, and infections, as well as an MRI of her brain—to make sure that we were not missing anything treatable. I also arranged a spinal tap, which involves putting a small needle into the bottom of the patient's spine to collect a sample of the fluid that lies around the brain. If these tests did not reveal evidence of strokes, a brain tumor, water on the brain (also called hydrocephalus), chronic meningitis, or another infection like syphilis or HIV, then we had to accept the diagnosis of Alzheimer's disease.

In patients with familial Alzheimer's disease, who make up only five to 10 percent of cases, it is possible to do DNA tests for genetic mutations that cause the disease. These tests prove positive in only a small proportion of cases, however. We have yet to find all the mutations and develop the appropriate DNA tests for every one. However, if we find a mutation in the patient, then we may offer genetic testing to his or her relatives. We particularly offer genetic counseling to young people who have not yet completed their families and may want to avoid giving birth to potentially affected children. It is essential to provide counseling before doing the test, because the implication of finding the mutation in a healthy person is that he or she may well develop the disease later.

The ApoE4 blood test can be done, but it does not indicate whether a person has Alzheimer's disease or might develop it. The presence of ApoE4 simply suggests that an individual is at a greater risk of developing the disease relative to other people.

## Treatment of Alzheimer's Disease

When the results of all the tests came in, I saw Mrs. Abramowitz and Betty in my office again. I told them that the tests had shown that indeed there were problems with her memory, and that I would arrange some treatment. Mrs. Abramowitz seemed satisfied, and I told her that she could go back into the waiting room while I wrote the prescription. I did this so that I could talk more with Betty about Alzheimer's disease, what she could expect, and what treatment we have available.

In writing prescriptions for patients with Alzheimer's disease, I caution family members like Betty not to expect too much. None of the drugs currently available cure or even arrest the progress of the disease. Still, some medications can improve the memory slightly. The neurons most severely damaged by Alzheimer's use a chemical called acetylcholine to send messages to each other. Medications that decrease the breakdown of acetylcholine help the memory a little. These medications include donepezil (Aricept®), rivastigmine (Exelon®), and galantamine (Razadyne®). Another medication that may slow the progress of Alzheimer's disease is memantine (Namenda®). This drug blocks a chemical in the brain called glutamate, too much of which damages neurons.

What we need are medications that prevent the precipitation of the abnormal proteins and preserve patients' synapses and neurons. Laboratory scientists have developed antibodies that remove precipitated beta-amyloid protein from the brains of mice genetically engineered to have a form of Alzheimer's disease. However, a trial of these antibodies in patients with Alzheimer's disease caused brain inflammation, a type of encephalitis. Eventually it may be possible to overcome this problem and remove beta-amyloid from the brains of patients. That might be the way to cure the disease.

## Course and Prognosis of Alzheimer's Disease

The first thing that goes in Alzheimer's patients is usually memory—most commonly, the ability to remember people's names. Amazingly, long-term memories remain relatively preserved until quite late in the process, and patients can often be engaged in discussions of times past with apparent clarity. The patient may seem quite normal for a few moments, but then he will lapse back into the dementia.

Insight and judgment begin to deteriorate when loss of memory and cognitive function become significant. At this stage, patients may become paranoid. For instance, they might forget where they put their keys and suspect that someone has stolen them. Eventually, patients may lose the ability to recognize their loved ones.

The rate at which these changes occur is surprisingly variable. Some patients become unable to look after themselves within a couple of years of their first symptoms. Others may remain able to live alone without help for five or more years. People with this slow progression are sometimes described as having minimal cognitive impairment. However, it seems to me more likely that they just have a slower form of Alzheimer's disease.

Betty brought her mother back to see me every three months and I was able to help her manage Mrs. Abramowitz as her condition gradually became worse. At first it was simply a matter of teaching her to use sticky notes all over the house—for example, "Turn off the stove," "Lock the front door," and "Take the house keys." But soon these tactics were not enough to keep her safe at home on her own. I recommended that Mrs. Abramowitz move in with Betty.

It was very difficult to persuade Mrs. Abramowitz to leave her house. In the end Betty had to employ a subterfuge. She told mother that her house needed to be fumigated for termites, so she would have to move out for a time. Mrs. Abramowitz accepted this explanation. Although she kept saying to Betty that it was time to go back home, she usually forgot about it a few minutes later.

Having her mother at home proved to be increasingly difficult for Betty. Mrs. Abramowitz began to need constant watching, and she had increasing outbursts of temper. Betty called me in tears one day and said that she couldn't stand it any longer. She told me that she felt very guilty, but she needed to move her mother into a chronic care facility. I made a visit to Betty's home and saw for myself all the problems she was having. Mrs. Abramowitz's room was a mess. A few weeks earlier she had caused a small fire after getting hold of a candle and matches. I said to Betty that she must not feel guilty; she had been an angel far beyond the powers of most families to cope with a patient at this stage of Alzheimer's disease.

The process of getting Mrs. Abramowitz to a nursing home was also difficult, but again, a subterfuge worked. We told her that she and Betty were going away for a little vacation, and Betty stayed with her mother in the nursing home for a few days until Mrs. Abramowitz had forgotten about living anywhere else.

The late stages of Alzheimer's disease are very sad, particularly for a patient's loved ones. The patient is totally out of contact with the world, and he often shouts or struggles uncontrollably. His ability to get around deteriorates, and he starts to have falls and to injure himself. Eventually he becomes bedridden, unable to feed himself, and doubly incontinent.

Over the next three years, I kept contact with Betty and occasionally visited Mrs. Abramowitz with her. In the first year Mrs. Abramowitz would sometimes recognize Betty, but at other times she would scream at her to go away: "You are not my daughter, and don't say you are!" This was very traumatic for Betty, though I helped her understand what was going on in her mother's failing brain. After two years, Mrs. Abramowitz became bedridden and incontinent. Betty was very distressed at this. She told me that she now understood mercy killing, which happens when a family member just cannot bear to see a loved one in such an awful condition.

Over the next six months, the nurses found it increasingly difficult to feed Mrs. Abramowitz, and eventually the nursing home doctor recommended to Betty that they put a feeding tube into her stomach. Betty called me about it. Was it the right thing to do? She reminded me that her mother had always feared ending up as a vegetable and had crafted a living will, with Betty appointed as her health care surrogate. I asked Betty if she had shown the forms to the doctor, and she said yes. She continued, "He told me that the PEG tube was the only way to keep Mother comfortable and to prevent her from choking or starving to death."

I went with Betty to meet the doctor and nurses at the nursing home so that we could all be on the same page. The nursing home staff knew that Mrs. Abramowitz was completely unaware of anything that was going on around her. We all agreed that Mrs. Abramowitz had not wanted to get to this state and had clearly indicated in her living will that she would not want it to be maintained. We further agreed that she would not have wanted a feeding tube. The nursing home staff would keep Mrs. Abramowitz comfortable by providing her with sedatives by rectal suppository and keeping her hydrated as much as possible through sips of water, but not forcing liquids or antibiotics. As her health care surrogate, Betty declined permission for a feeding tube. Mrs. Abramowitz died about a month later from pneumonia, which is sometimes called "the old person's friend."

In rare cases, Alzheimer's disease appears to stop progressing and the patient remains mildly demented but stable for several years. Stanislaw was a case in point. He had been a resistance fighter in the Warsaw Ghetto Uprising of 1943, in which 200,000 people died. He was one of the lucky few who escaped into the forests, joined the guerillas, and survived.

After the war Stanislaw moved to the United States, started a family, and eventually grew old. His wife and son brought him to me because his memory was deteriorating and he was becoming difficult to deal with. His first language was Yiddish, but he had learned enough English to get by in the United States. With the development of Alzheimer's disease, however, he had lost the ability to speak or understand English. All our communication took place through his son, who translated from Yiddish to English for me.

Stanislaw also complained bitterly of pain in his joints, particularly at night, when his shouting about the pain would wake everyone in the house. I gave him some anti-inflammatory medication in the hope of easing his pain and giving everyone a better night's sleep. This worked, and for several years the family would bring him back to see me regularly. At each visit, through his son, I would test Stanislaw's memory.

After a couple of years without any significant change in Stanislaw's cognitive abilities, his son asked me if this really was Alzheimer's disease. I told him that Stanislaw had all the symptoms of Alzheimer's disease and that none of the tests had suggested any other diagnosis. Stanislaw's memory remained stable for the next five years, and then he died of a heart attack. An autopsy was not done, so I will never know if he truly had Alzheimer's disease, but I always wondered if the anti-inflammatory medication was responsible for the arrest of his condition. Early research reports suggested that dementia was less frequent in patients taking anti-inflammatory drugs, but later trials have not been able to prove that these drugs are effective in treating Alzheimer's disease.

## Other Forms of Dementia

Good neurologists think about other conditions that can simulate Alzheimer's dementia, because some are treatable. These conditions include vitamin $B_{12}$ deficiency, thyroid hormone deficiency, syphilis, advanced AIDS, and some chronic infections in the fluid around the brain (called meningitis).

Another non-Alzheimer's dementia is called multi-infarct dementia. If someone has had two or three strokes and becomes demented after the last one, the diagnosis of multi-infarct dementia is easy. However, patients with multi-infarct dementia more commonly have a history of progressive loss of mental capacity, sometimes with periods of worsening and slight improvement. Scans of these patients' brains show evidence of several old strokes that went unnoticed because they occurred in a "silent" part of the brain—a part of the brain that is not as crucially important or eloquent as is the speech area in the left frontal lobe. Some of these noneloquent areas lie deep in the brain in areas like the thalamus and the basal ganglia, or in the white matter lying between those deep neuronal masses and the cerebral cortex. (I'll say more about this in the chapter on stroke.)

The presence of silent strokes in brain scans does not prove that the patient has multi-infarct dementia, since silent strokes can occur in an elderly person whose mind is very well-preserved. These silent strokes, whether the patient has dementia or not, are usually caused by damage to the small arteries deep in the brain, and they occur in people with chronic high blood pressure, diabetes, and high cholesterol. Because these conditions are treatable, to a large extent multi-infarct dementia is preventable.

A less common type of progressive dementia involves early loss of control of behavior and judgment but preservation of memory. Patients often become impulsive and childlike, and in the end they are completely disinhibited and uncontrollable. They might urinate anywhere when they have the urge or become sexually aggressive. This condition used to be called Pick's disease. Today we call it frontotemporal dementia because in MRI scans or at autopsy the brain shows atrophy concentrated in the frontal and temporal lobes.

There are several different causes of frontotemporal dementia, and researchers are still trying to understand them. Some cases run in families with known gene mutations, while many are sporadic—that is, there is no other case in the family. We now know that patients with amyotrophic lateral sclerosis (ALS, or Lou Gehrig's disease) frequently have some degree of frontotemporal dementia, especially if the disease begins to involve speech and swallowing (this is termed pseudobulbar involvement).

Another rare type of dementia is called diffuse Lewy body disease. In this condition, when the neurons of the cerebral cortex are examined under a microscope, they are seen to contain structures called Lewy bodies, named after the man who first described them. We know that Lewy bodies consist of precipitated proteins, but their exact composition is still being figured out. (In Parkinson's patients, Lewy bodies are found in dying neurons in the substantia nigra, an area at the base of the brain.) Patients with diffuse Lewy body disease typically begin to suffer hallucinations early in the course of a progressive dementia that fluctuates quite markedly from time to time. Many patients later develop parkinsonism. Drugs like haloperidol (Haldol®) can help control the hallucinations and psychosis, but they worsen the Parkinson-like symptoms.

A particularly dreaded though rare form of dementia is Creutzfeldt-Jakob disease (CJD), named after two German neurologists who first described the condition. This is a rapidly progressive dementia associated with jerks of the limbs, called myoclonus, and seizures. Death usually occurs within three to twenty-four months of the onset of symptoms. The disease tends to involve mature adults and is rare. The number of cases diagnosed in the United States each year amounts to about one in a million. At present there is no known treatment. CJD became famous when cases were discovered to arise from eating cattle affected by mad cow disease. This particular type, a rather slower form of the disease known medically as new variant Creutzfeldt-Jakob disease (nvCJD), tends to affect younger people.

CJD is a slow virus disease. Standard viruses are made of either DNA or RNA, usually wrapped in a protein coat. The virus of mad cow disease and CJD contains neither DNA nor RNA; it is composed of pure protein. It took many years for the scientific community to accept this, and in 1997 Stanley Prusiner was awarded the Nobel Prize in Physiology and Medicine for his work on what are now called prions.

The brains of normal humans and animals make prion protein, but what it is used for is still unknown. This normal protein is soluble, but it is somewhat unstable and liable to precipitate and become insoluble. It precipitates without any change in its chemical composition in a process that is much like the crystallization of a supersaturated solution of common salt that occurs when a crystal of salt is dropped into it.

People who have a mutation of the prion protein gene may develop CJD because the mutant protein is even more liable to precipitate than normal prion protein. Additionally, a person whose brain is exposed to the crystallized prion protein is very likely to develop CJD. This may happen to patients who receive grafts of a cornea or dura (brain-covering membrane) taken from cadavers who had CJD, unbeknownst to doctors. The disease may also develop in patients who receive human growth hormone prepared from pituitary glands of CJD patients.

One treatable form of dementia is normal pressure hydrocephalus (NPH, also called water on the brain). A person with this condition typically has a triad of symptoms: deterioration of mental capacity (though not specifically memory at the beginning), difficulty walking, and urinary incontinence. The patient's MRI shows enlargement of the cavities of the brain, called the ventricles, due to back pressure from partial blockage of the drainage of the CSF (cerebrospinal fluid) from the head. A relatively minor neurosurgical procedure can drain the CSF and thereby allow the ventricles to return to a more normal size. This reduces the pressure on the brain and improves the patient's problems.

A sixty-seven-year-old family doctor came to see me because of deterioration in his ability to walk. He was having difficulty taking care of his patients and had taken leave from his practice the previous month. When I asked if he was wetting himself, he admitted that this was happening increasingly. I told him that I thought he had NPH, and the MRI proved me right. Within a month of the neurosurgical operation, he was walking normally, had no urinary incontinence, and was back to seeing patients. In fact, he kept sending me all his difficult patients, whether they had a neurological problem or not, telling them, "You have to go to see Dr. Bradley. He will figure out what is wrong with you!"

## Chapter 3

# Stroke

A lbert was fifty-five. He worked in construction and was a bull of a man, but he did not take care of himself properly. He was 30 pounds overweight and drank a six-pack of beer every night. He had smoked two packs of cigarettes a day for forty years and refused to give them up, despite knowing the risks. He said that his father had smoked all his life and had lived to age eighty, so why should he quit? Albert also had high blood pressure, but since every one of the medications his doctor prescribed made him feel weak and dizzy, he refused treatment.

A week before Albert came into our emergency department with a full-blown stroke, on an evening that was no different from any other, he had a few beers and fell asleep in front of the TV. When he awoke and got up to go to the bathroom, he fell; his left leg would not work. His left arm also felt heavy. He figured he must have slept awkwardly, and he called to his wife to help him to bed. In the morning he was fine again, and he decided to forget about it. He did not know it at the time, but this was a warning attack, sometimes called a transient ischemic attack (TIA), indicating that he might soon have a more severe stroke.

The night Albert was stricken, a week later, he was having dinner with his wife when he suddenly keeled over and fell off his chair.

His wife was terrified. She called 911, and the ambulance arrived ten minutes later. The emergency medical technicians (EMTs) put him on a gurney and rushed him to our hospital. They called ahead to let our emergency department staff know that they were bringing in a patient with a brain attack. This is the term now used by neurologists and emergency doctors to make everyone aware of the urgency of getting a stroke patient to the hospital for treatment.

Albert was rushed into the triage area, where one of my residents, Dr. Cruz, was waiting to do a quick examination. He determined that Albert had paralysis of his left arm and leg, and weakness of the left side of Albert's face was evident when Dr. Cruz asked him to smile. His speech and vision seemed normal. Dr. Cruz asked Albert and his wife when the stroke had begun, and they confirmed that it had happened less than thirty minutes earlier.

Dr. Cruz immediately called the acute brain attack team, took some blood tests, and rushed Albert to the computerized tomography (CT) scanner. Ten minutes later Dr. Cruz looked at the scan and saw that Albert's brain looked normal, with no hemorrhage or swelling on the right side, which was where he knew the stroke was located. The stroke was probably caused by a sudden obstruction of the internal carotid artery—the main artery going to the right side of the brain. The normal CT scan meant that Albert had reached hospital before any irreparable damage to the brain had occurred.

Dr. Cruz took Albert from the CT scanner to the special annex of the emergency department devoted to the ultra-acute treatment of stokes and heart attacks. He already had an intravenous drip running, and now Dr. Cruz wrote a prescription for intravenous tPA (the chemical name is tissue plasminogen activator) to treat the clot that was blocking the right internal carotid artery. This drug, often called the "clot buster," is an enzyme that dissolves fibrin, a protein that holds a clot together. Once the fibrin is dissolved, the clot breaks up, and blood flow can return to the brain. tPA works best if it is given very early after the onset of a stroke; the "magic window" for tPA treatment is about three hours—hence the urgency with which the medical community regards a brain attack.

## Tests Used in the Diagnosis of Stroke

Exactly how doctors investigate the cause of a stroke depends on how soon they see the patient after the onset of symptoms. In Albert's case, he was within the "magic window," and he received the established emergency investigations for a brain attack.

Albert had blood tests to make sure that there was no problem of excessive blood clotting or signs of inflammation, which might have suggested that he was suffering from arteritis (inflammation of the wall of the carotid and other arteries) that can cause the artery to be blocked off. The tests also checked all his other systems to make sure he did not have diabetes, kidney failure, anemia, high cholesterol, or any other condition that the doctors would need to know about when planning his treatment.

While these tests were running in the lab, Albert was already having the CT scan of his brain. The CT scanner, which first came into clinical use in the early 1970s, gives us a dramatically effective way to look inside the skull at the brain. The scanner works in the following way. A thin pencil of X-rays is shone from one side of the skull to the other, where it is received by a small X-ray detector. If the X-ray beam goes through dense brain tissue, few of the X-rays will reach the detector; where the brain tissue is not dense, more X-rays will reach the detector. The X-ray generator moves a few degrees at a time in a circle around the head of the patient and keeps repeating the process. This goes on very rapidly until the generator has circled the head completely. Then the generator shifts up a half a centimeter and repeats the process. In this way, the machine takes a series of X-ray slices of the whole head. The results from the detectors are stored in a computer.

Now comes the interesting part. Via amazingly complex calculations done at the speed of light, the computer converts all the data from the detectors into a picture of the density of the brain in each tiny area. These pictures are presented as a series of slices through the brain, sometimes called tomograms, which is why the machine is called a computer tomography scanner.

If Albert had suffered a brain hemorrhage, the blood that leaked into the brain would have shown up as a dense white mass on the CT scan. On the other hand, if the loss of blood supply to the right side of his brain had gone on for an hour or more, the CT scan would have shown that the damaged area of brain was less dense than normal and swollen. This would have indicated that the brain had suffered irreparable damage, for which the medical term is *infarction*.

Another form of brain imaging, the MRI scan, is produced in a similar way to the CT scan, but magnetic waves are sent through the brain rather than X-rays. MRI scans are much more informative than CT scans; they can even be used to determine whether the brain tissue is still alive or dead. However, MRI scans take longer than the fastest CT scans. Therefore, they are not so helpful in the emergency situation of investigating a patient with an acute brain attack.

Albert had two other tests after he started getting the tPA intravenously. One was a carotid artery ultrasound/Doppler study, and the other was an electrocardiogram (EKG).

The technician doing the carotid artery ultrasound/Doppler study put an ultrasound probe on Albert's neck. This type of probe works like a sonar submarine detector. He found that atheroma (also called plaque) was narrowing the right internal carotid artery in Albert's neck, and that there was a clot on the rough area of the plaque. The narrowing, or stenosis, appeared to be critical, meaning that the channel in the middle of the artery had narrowed to about 5 percent of its normal size.

The technician then put the probe over Albert's right temple to determine if the blood was flowing in the correct direction in the right middle cerebral artery. This is called a transcranial Doppler study. Normally, the blood in the anterior cerebral artery flows away from the ultrasound probe, but with a critical stenosis of the right carotid artery in the neck, as in Albert's case, the direction of flow is reversed because blood is coming from the left internal carotid artery via connections between vessels at the base of the brain. While doing the transcranial Doppler study, the technician detected little clots or emboli passing across the ultrasound beam. Each one produced a short sharp noise called a high-intensity transient, or HIT. Because atheroma had severely narrowed the right carotid artery in Albert's neck, the clots were believed to be coming from there, though theoretically they could have been coming from the heart.

Other technicians performed an EKG to see if Albert had suffered a silent heart attack or if he had an abnormal heart rhythm, such as atrial fibrillation. Either of these conditions could have caused the blood in the heart to clot, and a small part of this clot might have broken off and flipped into one of the arteries going to the brain, thus producing the stroke. Albert's EKG was normal, however. Had there been any reason to think that his heart was responsible for the stroke, additional tests such as an echocardiogram would have been done.

I came on the scene at this time and discussed with Dr. Cruz what more we should do. In order to decide if Albert needed surgery to open up the artery and take out the plaque, we needed to know exactly how severe the narrowing of the right internal carotid artery was. One option was a special MRI scan called an MR angiogram (MRA), which shows the larger arteries in the neck and brain. Another choice was a catheter angiogram, in which a fine plastic tube (catheter) is threaded through a needle in the femoral artery in the groin and steered through the aorta (the body's main artery) into the arteries in the neck. Dye that can be seen on X-rays is injected through this catheter to reveal the state of the arteries supplying the brain. Since the MRA is almost as good as a catheter angiogram for showing the arteries, and is noninvasive and hence would be less uncomfortable and risky for Albert, we decided to do an MRA.

## What Is a Stroke?

A stroke is like a heart attack, but it affects the brain rather than the heart. For this reason, we now call an acute stroke a brain attack. The medical term for a stroke is a cerebral vascular accident (CVA). A stroke is a major life-altering event. Stroke is the third most common cause of death in developed countries like the United States and the most common cause of severe disability. Three-quarters of a million Americans suffer a stroke each year. One-fifth of them die of the stroke, and at least one-third remain permanently disabled. Cerebral vascular disease costs the U.S. health care system an estimated $60 billion each year.

Strokes are caused by one of two problems that may develop in the arteries of the brain. One is blockage of the arteries, and the other is a rupture that allows a hemorrhage to occur. Neurologists sometimes irreverently apply plumbing terms to these problems—*plugs* and *leaks*.

## Plugs

Plugs occur when a brain artery becomes blocked, thus cutting off blood to the part of the brain that it supplies. The technical term for blockage of the artery is cerebral thrombosis and the term for the resultant damage to the brain is cerebral ischemia. Of all the body's cells, neurons are the most vulnerable to loss of blood supply. Skin and bone cells can live for many hours without blood, but neurons require a continuous supply of oxygen and glucose, and they will die if their blood supply is cut off for just a few minutes.

Different neurons have different levels of vulnerability to loss of the blood supply. Those in the spinal cord are able to survive longest (twenty minutes), and those in the brain stem can survive for ten minutes, while neurons in the hippocampus and cerebral cortex last only five minutes without blood. If the blood supply to an area of the brain is blocked for a prolonged period—several hours or more—then both the neurons and their supporting cells, called glia, die, and the patient suffers what is called a cerebral infarction.

One cause of blockage of an artery supplying the brain is an embolus. This is the medical term for something that gets wedged in the artery and blocks it. In most cases, the embolus is a piece of a blood clot. A common site for an embolus to wedge is in the middle cerebral artery, where it branches into two smaller arteries. An embolus causes an ultrarapid onset of a stroke. One minute the patient is fine, and the next moment he has a severe paralysis of the opposite side of the body.

An embolus commonly comes from a clot in one of four locations. One is plaque in the wall of the aorta; blood clots easily on the plaque's rough surface. Another is plaque in the internal carotid artery in the neck, as in Albert's case. Another location is a clot inside the heart. This can be caused by atrial fibrillation (which causes blood pools in the quivering upper chambers of the heart to clot), or it can happen after a heart attack, when a clot forms on the dead tissue in the cavity of the heart. Yet another source is a clot in a leg vein (a deep vein thrombosis). You may be asking yourself, How can a clot in the veins travel to the brain, since the veins return blood to the right side of the heart to be pumped to the lungs? Well, about 25 percent of people have a hole in the heart that goes from the right (venous) side to the left (arterial) side. This hole in the heart—called a patent foramen ovale—should have closed soon after birth but didn't, and it provides a pathway for clots to pass from the veins into the arteries of the brain.

Another cause of stroke is cerebral thrombosis. This happens when a clot forms on plaque in the wall of an artery going to the brain, thus blocking the artery. Sometimes the plaque may severely narrow the channel through the artery without totally blocking it. Some blood may get through, but not enough. This occurred in Albert's situation; the channel was down to less than 5 percent of its normal size. Because the plaque and the clot develop slowly, the resulting stroke may gradually worsen over several hours.

Cerebral embolus and cerebral thrombosis are not totally different. Both may result from plaque in the arteries. As we can see from Albert's case, in which the internal carotid artery was not completely obstructed, little clots may break off and wedge in a small artery, but because they are soft they may quickly dissolve. The loss of blood supply to the small area of brain is therefore very transient, and no death of neurons results. This kind of ministroke is called a transient ischemic attack (TIA). By definition the stroke symptoms last very briefly—certainly less than twenty-four hours—and clear up completely. Albert had experienced such a TIA a week before he suffered his disastrous stroke.

Inflammation in the wall of a major cerebral artery—due, for instance, to temporal arteritis, a condition that causes bad headaches in the elderly—can also cause a clot to form, to block the artery wall, and thus to produce a stroke. A cause of stroke that can occur in young, active people is a tear in the lining of an artery wall that allows blood to make its way under the vessel lining and even to push the artery wall inward. We call this an arterial dissection, and it can lead to enough obstruction to cause a stroke.

A different type of blockage that can cause a ministroke occurs in the very small arteries that lie deep in the substance of the brain. Blockage of these small arteries is usually caused by damage to the arterial wall resulting from chronic high blood pressure and diabetes. The resulting ministroke destroys a small volume of brain tissue and leaves a small hole in the brain, called a lacune. Many lacunes are detected only by brain imaging studies because they occur in "silent areas" of the brain. Hence, many ministrokes occur without any corresponding symptoms.

*Leaks*

Leaks, the other main cause of strokes, occur when a blood vessel ruptures into either the brain or the subarachnoid space that lies around the brain. Blood rupturing into the brain—the medical term is intracerebral hemorrhage—destroys brain tissue and increases the pressure inside the head. On the other hand, blood rupturing into the space around the brain that contains cerebrospinal fluid—this is called a subarachnoid hemorrhage—does not immediately destroy brain tissue but does instantaneously raise the pressure inside the head to the level of the arterial blood pressure. The patient immediately becomes unconscious because the high pressure prevents blood from getting to the brain through its arteries. Blood in the subarachnoid space is very irritating. It produces a picture like meningitis—severe headache, fever, and stiff neck.

In the past—and even today, in situations where medical care is suboptimal, as in poorer areas of the United States and in many developing countries—cerebral hemorrhage resulting from high blood pressure is the most common cause of stroke. The ancient Greeks recognized two conditions that could suddenly strike down a person "like a bolt from the Gods": epilepsy and stroke. In places where patients receive good treatment for their hypertension, the frequency of hemorrhagic strokes has decreased. Now those areas see more patients with strokes caused by blockage of arteries (cerebral infarction or thrombosis).

The most common and most damaging cause of bleeding into the brain is chronic high blood pressure (hypertension). This condition can cause little bulges or blowouts to form on tiny blood vessels deep in the brain. These bulges are called Charcot-Bouchard aneurysms. One of these tiny aneurysms may suddenly rupture when the blood pressure rises rapidly, as with anger, sexual intercourse, or even straining on the toilet. As a result, blood under high pressure is forced into the brain substance, thus producing an intracerebral hemorrhage. If the back pressure from the brain tissue is sufficient, the bleeding will stop and the patient will survive, but usually he will be left with severe neurological damage. If the bleeding continues, the patient is likely to die.

A subarachnoid hemorrhage frequently results from the rupture of a cerebral aneurysm—a blowout on one of the larger arteries at the base of the brain. Most cerebral aneurysms are congenital, meaning that the patient was born with a weakness of the arterial wall that allowed it to gradually give way and produce the blowout. These aneurysms usually cause no symptoms unless they rupture. Only one in ten cerebral aneurysms ruptures, and most never cause symptoms. Unruptured aneurysms are relatively common findings on imaging studies of the intracranial blood vessels.

Aneurysms may make their presence known in a most dramatic fashion by suddenly rupturing after the wall of the aneurysm becomes thinner and suddenly gives way. Blood at arterial pressure then rushes out into the subarachnoid space around the brain, and the patient experiences a sudden high pressure inside her head. Patients say this feels like they have been hit on the head with a hammer to produce a "10 out of 10" headache. Pain in the head is often accompanied by nausea and vomiting. The patient may lose consciousness because the pressure inside her skull is so high that it prevents blood from entering the capillaries and providing oxygen to the brain.

An aneurysm that ruptures is usually on one of the arteries at the base of the brain, but in rare cases it may be on an artery on the spinal cord. One of my patients suffered a spinal subarachnoid hemorrhage when he was going down an escalator. Feeling as though he had been kicked in the back, he turned around and punched the man who was on the step behind him.

Subarachnoid hemorrhage caused by an aneurysm rupturing is extremely serious. One-third of patients die as a result of the acute attack, and up to half the patients who survive it are left with significant neurological damage, such as hemiparesis (weakness down one side of the body). A small number of patients with subarachnoid hemorrhage have family members who experienced the same condition. In that case, it is likely that they have a familial tendency to develop cerebral aneurysms. All the relatives may be offered a magnetic resonance angiogram (MRA) to show the arteries inside the skull and thus to pick up aneurysms before they rupture. However, the identification of a cerebral aneurysm presents any patient with a difficult decision: Do I have the aneurysm dealt with, or do I leave it? I will discuss this shortly.

Sometimes an area of weakness of a congenital arteriovenous malformation (AVM) may cause an intracranial hemorrhage, either a subarachnoid or an intracerebral bleed. People may be born with an AVM—a tangle of blood vessels formed where there is an abnormal connection between the brain's arteries and veins. The blood vessels in an AVM are very fragile and rupture easily, but the blood vessels are often not arteries, and therefore the hemorrhage is less severe than those due to other causes.

# Clinical Features of Stroke and Their Causes

The location of the stroke is of great importance in terms of the patient's symptoms and the extent of his disability. For instance, Albert was lucky that the stroke was on the right side of his brain. Had it been on the left side, he would have been unable to speak. As I described in Chapter 1, for most people, production of speech is located in the part of the left frontal lobe of the brain called Broca's area, lying just under the left temple. Damage to the area served by the left middle cerebral artery also may cause weakness of the right face and arm. Loss of the ability to produce words and sentences is called motor aphasia. Many aphasic patients can understand what is said to them but are unable to reply.

A different form of speech and language disturbance may result from a stroke in the left posterior temporal area, the part of the brain that lies just above the left ear called Wernicke's area. As I described in the Chapter 1 section about the left cerebral hemisphere, damage to this area can cause sensory aphasia, in which the patient's speech is unintelligible, or "word salad."

A stroke that damages all the nerve fibers going from the motor cortex to the corticospinal (pyramidal) tracts will cause paralysis of the opposite arm, leg, and face. This is because the brain is "crossed": one side of the cerebral cortex relates to the opposite side of the body. This paralysis is called a complete hemiplegia. However, if the area affected by the stroke is smaller—for instance, if the middle cerebral artery is blocked—then only the arm and face become paralyzed; the leg is unaffected because it is the anterior cerebral artery that supplies the leg area of the cerebral cortex. Conversely, blockage of an anterior cerebral artery produces paralysis of the opposite leg but spares the arm and face.

Blockage of one posterior cerebral artery at the back of the brain may produce loss of vision in the opposite half of the visual field. The patient becomes unable to see something on the side opposite the stroke, unless he turns his head to look straight at it.

If the basilar artery, which lies just in front of the brain stem deep at the back of the skull, becomes blocked, then the stroke will damage the brain stem. This is the part of the brain through which all nerve fibers run to and from the brain, and where consciousness is located. A patient with a brain stem stroke usually becomes suddenly unconscious and develops quadriplegia—complete paralysis of all four limbs.

Occasionally, a patient who has had a brain stem stroke will recover consciousness but remain "locked in"—that is, he is awake but unable to communicate, to move a limb, or even to move his face, though usually his eye movements are left intact. Neurologists aware of this possibility can usually determine if the patient is in this locked-in state by asking the patient to move his eyes, for this is often the only voluntary movement that the patient retains. Through eye movements, doctors can communicate with "locked-in" patients and determine that they are alert and aware of what is happening around them. This is a pretty terrifying condition, and few patients survive or make any significant recovery. The dramatic movie, *The Diving Bell and the Butterfly*, was based on the book by Jean-Dominique Bauby, who suffered such a stroke and dictated the text by blinking, his only voluntary movement.

Blockage of a small artery deep in the brain may produce a lacune. If this destroys the part of the deep white matter of the brain in an area termed the internal capsule, where all the nerve fibers running to and from the brain are concentrated, the result may be paralysis or partial loss of sensation in the face, arm, and leg on the opposite side of the body. Because a lacune is very small, it may affect movement without interfering with sensation, or vice versa. It may even affect the nerve fibers going to only one limb.

We tend to think that every part of the brain is essential. Surprisingly, large areas, even up to the size of a quarter, may be damaged by a stroke without the patient suffering any obvious neurological effect. It is not unusual for the MRI of a patient who has just suffered a stroke to show several previous strokes that caused the patient no symptoms. The explanation is that there are multiple redundancies of many parts of the brain, and some areas lack the eloquence that is characteristic of the speech and motor areas.

A patient's symptoms and level of disability also depend on the amount of brain tissue damaged by the stroke. Because a lacune is small, its effects may resolve completely in a few days. On the other hand, if a large area of the cerebral cortex dies from oxygen starvation, there will be very little recovery of function. One good feature of the brain's arterial blood supply is that it has many connections, called anastomoses, between major arteries. For instance, the middle cerebral artery connects with the anterior and posterior cerebral arteries on the same side of the brain. These connections, called collateral blood supply, can save an area of brain from being completely destroyed. There are also connections within the skull between the arteries on the two sides of the brain. I once cared for a patient who had complete blockage of all four main arteries supplying the brain, but he was kept alive by anastomoses between the external carotid artery branches in his scalp and the intracranial arteries.

Also crucial with regard to symptoms and disability is the duration of loss of blood supply. If an important area of brain lacks its blood supply for several hours, the stroke will be severe. If the obstruction of the artery lasts only a minute or two, as with a small embolus, then the consequent loss of neurological function will be temporary. A stroke that lasts less than twenty-four hours and is followed by complete recovery is called a TIA.

TIAs can foreshadow a major stroke, however, and therefore they need to be investigated urgently. We saw in the case of Albert, who had an episode of weakness in his left leg and arm a week before his major stroke. When I questioned him later, he admitted that he had been having strange episodes of blurred vision for a couple of months. I asked if he knew which eye had been affected. He told me that he knew it was the right, because when he had covered the left eye during these spells, he had found he could not see anything with the right eye. Doctors call these attacks of loss of vision in one eye amaurosis fugax, which means "fleeting loss of vision." In Albert's case they occurred when little clots broke off from the plaque of atheroma in his right internal carotid artery and temporarily blocked the blood supply to his right eye. If Albert had seen a neurologist about these TIAs, he probably would have avoided the major stroke.

## Treatment and Prognosis of Stroke

The acute brain attack program that we used for Albert was very successful. Three hours after we started the tPA, he got some movement back in his left leg. Over the next two days, his left hemiplegia completely resolved. We did another MRA and found that, despite tPA treatment, the right internal carotid artery was still 80 percent narrowed by plaque. We referred him to the neurosurgeon, who opened up the artery and removed the plaque that was causing the narrowing. The operation was uneventful, and Albert walked out of the hospital six days after his stroke.

There is only a small window of opportunity to prevent complete death of the area of the brain affected by a stroke. The earlier the tPA treatment is started, the better. The guidelines recommend that treatment should not be given if the stroke has been present for more than three hours because it can cause hemorrhage into the already-damaged brain after that time.

An acute brain attack team consists of neurologists, emergency department physicians, neuroradiologists, and neurosurgeons. The team must be able to complete their investigations and initiate treatment within minutes of the patient's admittance to the hospital. They have to be skilled in the intricacies of all the necessary techniques that I have described, and they must be available around the clock. A full brain attack team is expensive to maintain and is available in relatively few hospitals, mainly those associated with medical schools. The team needs to be very experienced because the wrong decision can result in disaster. However, when the arterial blockage is successfully relieved it is wonderful to behold the almost miraculous return of function to paralyzed limbs, as in Albert's case, or the recovery of speech in someone who was totally aphasic.

## Treating the completed stroke

Treatment of a completed stroke is currently all we have to offer patients who come to the hospital many hours or even days after the stroke began. Theoretically, drugs called neuroprotective agents could keep injured neurons alive, but so far no such drug has proved to be effective. The keystones of good medical treatment of stroke are preventing fever, keeping the blood sugar levels within normal range in patients with diabetes, and maintaining the blood pressure at correct levels. The reason for this is that anything that upsets the biochemistry of the already-injured brain is going to increase the amount of tissue damage.

The guideline for control of blood pressure is "not too high, not too low, but just right." If a patient's blood pressure is reduced too much, the collateral blood supply from the other arteries that are trying to keep the ischemic brain alive will be reduced, with negative effects on the stroke. Generally we try to avoid blood pressure lower than about 150/90. In patients like Albert, who have chronic hypertension, blood pressure should not be brought to normal levels (120/80), since the brain and its blood vessels have become used to living on high blood pressure.

## Preventing further strokes

Prevention of future problems is an essential part of the treatment of any stroke patient. This includes investigating the stroke's cause to ensure that the same thing will not happen again. If doctors find a clot in the heart or in the arteries of the neck, then blood-thinning drugs like heparin and Coumadin may be used to prevent further clots. If there is a hole in the heart, a device like a tiny umbrella can be put into the heart to close the hole.

Albert was a typical stroke victim. He was overweight, he smoked, and he did not treat his high blood pressure. We also found that he had high cholesterol and lipids in his blood. We needed to treat all of these stroke risk factors in order to prevent him from having another stroke. I explained to Albert that unless he took an active role in changing his lifestyle by giving up smoking, losing some weight, and letting us treat his high blood pressure and cholesterol, he would likely either die of a heart attack or have another severe stroke within two years. And a second stroke would likely kill him or render him permanently disabled. We kept a close watch on him with his internist, and I am happy to report that he responded to our advice.

## Treatment of subarachnoid hemorrhage and intracranial aneurysms

A patient who has had a subarachnoid hemorrhage in the last twenty-four hours may be totally unconscious. On the other hand, he may be awake and alert but suffering from a bad headache. The immediate symptoms depend on how much blood leaked out of the burst aneurysm. A great deal of research on how best to treat the hemorrhage itself has shown that, as with an acute stroke, good intensive care treatment is the best. We keep the blood pressure to normal levels of 120/80 and prevent blood sugar levels and fever from getting high. If the patient wakes up from a severe subarachnoid hemorrhage, he generally will not have a severe neurological problem of the type seen in patients who have a major stroke.

Information from many studies of patients with subarachnoid hemorrhage indicates that the earlier the aneurysm is closed off, the better the outcome for the patient. This is because once an aneurysm has burst, it is very likely to do so again within a short time, often with fatal results. Open neurosurgical operations may be used to put a clip on an aneurysm, thus preventing blood under high arterial pressure from reaching it. Alternatively, an endovascular procedure, done with a catheter introduced through the femoral artery in the leg and guided

16

up to the aneurysm, can fill the aneurysm with wire or glue to block it off internally.

A patient who has already survived a subarachnoid hemorrhage really has no choice but to undergo one of these procedures; there is too much danger of the aneurysm rupturing again. A person who is found to have an unruptured aneurysm is on the horns of a dilemma. The procedures that close the aneurysm are risky, yet a subarachnoid hemorrhage from a ruptured aneurysm has a real chance of being devastating. The patient should make this decision in consultation with an experienced neurosurgeon. It should be based on the details of the aneurysm and the estimated risks of the recommended procedure.

A few aneurysms grow to a very large size. They put pressure on the brain and cause symptoms such as hemiparesis. These giant aneurysms rupture only rarely, but there is no guarantee. Many neurosurgeons try to block off the aneurysm by using one of the two procedures mentioned for ruptured aneurysms.

### Rehabilitation of a completed stroke

It is important to focus on rehabilitation after a patient suffers a stroke. Albert did not need rehabilitation because he made a complete recovery, but Manuel was not so lucky.

At sixty-four, Manuel was a right-handed Hispanic man and an illegal immigrant. He had no health insurance and had not seen a doctor for ten years. One Saturday evening, he noticed that his right arm was weak. He thought it might be a pinched nerve. Manuel went to sleep, but when he got out of bed the next morning he fell because his right leg would not work properly. That day he stayed in bed, but the following morning the weakness was worse and he was having difficulty speaking. On Tuesday, his wife called an ambulance because she could not take care of him.

When my neurology team and I examined Manuel, he was totally unable to move his right arm and leg. The lower part of the right side of his face was weak, and he could not say a word. However, he seemed to understand everything we said to him in Spanish. The MRI scan showed that the tissue in the area of the brain supplied by the left middle cerebral artery was dead (we call this a completed stroke). We also found that he had chronic hypertension and high cholesterol.

We admitted Manuel to hospital and started to treat the hypertension and high cholesterol. The nurses made sure that he was turned every two hours to prevent bedsores and pneumonia. They fitted him with an external condom catheter to prevent urine from leaking into the bed. The rehabilitation team initiated physical, occupational, and speech therapy. Though Manuel had no insurance, our county hospital provided him with all needed medical care. After a week, we transferred him to the subacute rehabilitation service, where he began to get out of bed. Four weeks later Manuel was transferred to a chronic care facility, where he continued rehabilitation.

In recent animal research and investigation of patients recovering from a stroke, techniques such as functional MRI have shown that new areas of the brain can take over the functions lost by a brain damaged in a stroke. Surviving neurons are capable of sending new connections to other surviving neurons, and they can be stimulated to do so more fully with newer rehabilitation techniques. Neurological rehabilitation is a very slow process, however. It requires great patience and perseverance on the part of the patient and family, as well as the doctor and therapists.

A week after Manuel had his stroke, the rehab nurses saw him move his right arm for the first time when he yawned. But this was a reflex; when the nurses asked him to move his right arm voluntarily, he could not do it. The stroke had destroyed the pathway for voluntary movement that ran from the motor area of his left cerebral cortex to his right arm, but it had not affected the involuntary pathways. Stretching one's arm is a reflex movement that goes along with a yawn. Over the next few months, the therapists were able to teach Miguel to use those involuntary pathways to move his right arm.

A few weeks later, Manuel was sitting in a chair at the chronic care facility when a nurse accidentally ran a cart over his foot. Although he had not said a word since the stroke, he suddenly let out a string of expletives. The nurse was shocked, particularly since immediately afterward Manuel was unable to tell her what she had done to cause this outburst. This involuntary moment of speech was similar to the arm movement accompanying Manuel's yawn. The speech therapist was happy to hear about it, because it meant that she could start training him to speak again.

Manuel made an incomplete recovery from his stroke, and he was never able to work again. After a month he began to get some voluntary movement back in his right leg, and eventually he learned to walk with a cane. The leg was very stiff, and he swung it out when he walked. Doctors call this a spastic gait. His right arm never really improved; it remained bent at the elbow and tucked into his chest. He could use it to hold something against his chest but not to do much else. His speech never returned to normal, but eventually he was able to say what he wanted: "Get ... box." "Go ... toilet." "Where daughter ... Tina?" Most of the recovery after a severe stroke happens within the first six months, but as Manuel's case illustrates, further recovery may continue for one or two years.

Two separate symptoms may affect people who suffer a left hemiplegia due to a stroke of the right cerebral cortex. One is depression, and treatment with antidepressant medications and counseling can be of great help. The other symptom is what neurologists call neglect. This symptom causes patients to lose awareness of the left side of their body, often coupled with loss of awareness of the left side of the world. These patients may even lose awareness that there is anything wrong with their left-hand paralyzed limbs. Neurologists call this condition anosognosia.

## Other Types of Stroke

Strokes in people under the age of forty-five often result from conditions other than hypertension and hardening of the arteries, which are the common causes of stroke in the elderly. As I have mentioned, inflammation of the arteries supplying the brain and tears in an artery wall may cause stroke in young people. But cardiac sources of emboli, including a hole in the heart, are the most common causes of stroke in this age group. Various coagulation disorders of the blood may also lead to strokes, particularly the disorders that lead to excessive clotting. Women who take oral contraceptives and continue to smoke are at increased risk of stroke, too.

In very rare cases, migraines are responsible for strokes in young people. Migraine headaches cause spasm of the cerebral arteries, and some medications used to break a migraine attack cause arteries to contract even more, thus decreasing the blood supply to the brain. In addition, in several rare conditions, migraine and stroke tend to occur in the same patient. One is a mitochondrial disease named MELAS, which stands for mitochondrial encephalomyopathy, lactic acidosis, and stroke. (Mitochondria are the minute energy factories in every cell.) Another condition that causes strokes that run in families is called CADASIL, short for cerebral autosomal dominant arteriopathy with subcortical infarcts and leukoencephalopathy.

Inherited diseases of the arteries are rare causes of strokes in young people. Some years ago, I consulted with a twenty-four-year-old man after his third stroke in five years. Looking in his eyes with an ophthalmoscope, I saw a number of streaks of darker color going across his normal pink retina. These are called angioid streaks, and they told me that he had Ehlers-Danlos syndrome. This is a rare inherited abnormality of collagen, the tough fibrous material that provides the strength of most tissues and scars. This disease weakens the collagen at the back of the eye and in the blood vessels. The weakened blood vessels tear easily and may cause a stroke. Patients with this syndrome have abnormally lax joints and skin. I was able to confirm the diagnosis by bending the young patient's fingers back onto his wrist, showing the extreme flexibility of his joints that caused him no pain. Unfortunately, there is still no treatment for Ehlers-Danlos syndrome.

It's also important to remember that not everything that looks like a stroke actually is one. The following conditions may be mistaken for a stroke:

- a brain tumor
- a clot (subdural hematoma) between the covering of the brain (dura) and the subarachnoid space
- a seizure
- a faint
- a rhythm defect of the heart leading to a faint, which we call cardiogenic syncope
- hemiplegic migraine—a recurrent type of migraine in which each attack is associated with a temporary weakness of the limbs on one side

Global cerebral ischemia is the term given to damage to the brain that occurs if all its blood supply is cut off. Unlike a stroke, which damages a specific area of the brain, global cerebral ischemia affects all parts of the brain. The most common cause is cardiac arrest from a heart attack. If EMTs get to the patient in time, they can often get the heart beating again and prevent irreversible brain damage. If the heart was stopped for more than five minutes, however, the brain may suffer permanent damage (this is called anoxic brain damage or global cerebral ischemia). Similar global damage may follow carbon monoxide poisoning, which prevents the hemoglobin in the red cells from carrying oxygen from the lungs to the neurons.

Oxygen starvation affects some neurons more than others. The neurons of the cerebral cortex and hippocampus are particularly vulnerable. Patients who suffer global cerebral ischemia often remain unconscious for days and may wake up with memory problems, such as Korsakoff's syndrome. A few are left with severe damage to motor functions. I have a friend who was strangled and left for dead by a psychotic man she was interviewing for a newspaper article. She survived and recovered all her mental capacity, but the prolonged lack of oxygen to the motor centers of her brain left her severely spastic, with very stiff limbs and slowed movements. Despite this, she overcame her disabilities and became an Olympic sailing champion.

Another patient who suffered global cerebral anoxia was a newly retired doctor who moved into a new house with his wife in the middle of a New England winter. The builders had connected the flue from the boiler wrongly, and carbon monoxide slowly filled the house. Three days later, they were rescued and given emergency oxygen under high pressure in a hyperbaric chamber. Both the doctor and his wife remained in a coma for several days, though they survived. She eventually made a full recovery, but after a few weeks he quite quickly developed signs like those in Parkinson's disease, with very slow movements but little tremor. The carbon monoxide had destroyed the neurons in the doctor's basal ganglia, deep in the brain, causing a Parkinson-like condition.

Some patients who suffer global cerebral ischemia never regain useful brain function, and they remain in a persistent vegetative state for years. Perhaps the most famous case is Terri Schiavo, the young Florida housewife whose husband and family attracted national attention with their battle over withdrawing life support after Schiavo had been in that condition for more than a decade.

## Public Education about Stroke

More research is needed to find the best way to treat stroke, since tPA does not cure every patient and cannot be given once the three-hour window has passed. Other clot-busting drugs—and other ways of administering them, such as putting them directly into the blocked artery by means of an angiogram catheter—may turn out to be better than intravenous tPA. Treatments that are currently used for coronary artery disease of the heart are being studied for use in the treatment of blocked arteries in stroke patients. One technique is to insert instruments through an angiogram catheter to "roto-rooter" out the clot.

Another is to insert a rigid tube called a stent into an artery to open up a narrowed area.

There is hope for the future of stroke treatment. Scientists are researching ways of restoring neurological function lost to a stroke. Embryonic stem cell grafts may eventually be capable of producing neurons and glial cells that can connect and integrate into the existing neuronal circuits of the brain.

But while doctors and neuroscientists strive to find better ways to treat stroke, the most crucial thing we can do to alter the outcome of stroke is to educate the general public about brain attacks. At present only about 4 percent of stroke patients come into the emergency department within three hours of the onset of their stroke—that is, within the magic window when tPA can be given. Most patients with stroke symptoms go to bed and hope that they will be better in the morning. By then, it is too late to employ the acute brain attack program. We need people to respond to any symptoms that *might* be caused by a stroke, such as tingling or weakness in one limb, sudden onset of difficulty with speech, or vertigo. They should respond in exactly the same way that they would respond to chest pain: call an ambulance and get to the nearest hospital to have it checked out.

Fortunately, only a minority of people with these symptoms is actually having a stroke. This is both the good news and the bad news. The medical system would be overwhelmed if *everyone* with one of these symptoms went to an emergency department. Nevertheless, if we do not educate the general public about the need to seek medical attention urgently when these symptoms last for more than a few minutes, then we will never increase the proportion of stroke patients who walk out of the hospital cured.

## Chapter 4

# Epilepsy

Clint was fifteen when he had his first seizure. His parents were awakened by a loud cry coming from his bedroom. They rushed in and found him stretched out in the bed, stiff as a board, not breathing, and blue in the face. Almost immediately, he began thrashing around on the bed, started breathing and grunting, and became very red in the face. Thinking it was a nightmare, his father tried to wake him, but Clint did not respond. His father then tried to hold him down but found it almost impossible to control him because of the seemingly superhuman strength in Clint's arms and legs. The seizure went on for three minutes. Clint then quieted down, but his parents still could not wake him. Ten minutes later he started to come around, but he was drowsy and confused for over an hour. They also discovered that Clint had wet the bed, something he hadn't done since he was a baby. Clint complained that his tongue hurt, and they found that he had bitten it badly during the seizure.

Clint's mother had a brother with epilepsy, so she had recognized the telltale signs. Nevertheless, she had been terrified when they could not wake him and had called 911. By the time the EMTs arrived, Clint was awake. They wanted to take him to the emergency department of the nearest hospital. Clint's mother said she did not think he needed to go to hospital. Instead she decided to call me, because I was her brother's neurologist.

When I saw him the next morning, Clint was back to normal, except for his sore tongue and aching muscles. He remembered nothing from the time he went to sleep until the moment he awoke with his parents beside his bed and his mother crying.

When I examined Clint, I found that his nervous system was functioning normally. I arranged an EEG and an MRI scan of his brain. I told Clint and his parents that he probably had had a seizure resulting from a tendency that appeared to run in his mother's family. I recommended an anticonvulsant medication that Clint would take for three months. If he had no further seizures, I would stop the medication.

## What Is Epilepsy?

In ancient times, people with seizures were thought to be possessed by the gods, and so epilepsy was called "the sacred disease." Hippocrates, however, concluded that the disease arose from the brain. Aristotle was the first to connect epilepsy with genius, though we still do not know the reason for this association. More modern famous epilepsy sufferers (people who have recurrent seizures) were Van Gogh, Edward Lear, Dostoevsky, James Madison, and Richard Burton.

More than one in two hundred of the populations in developed countries, and three times that number in developing countries, suffer from epilepsy. In developing countries seizures are much more frequent because of the prevalence of infections and other conditions that damage the brain.

In a developed country like the United States, about 5 percent of the population has suffered one or two seizures in their lifetime (this is not enough seizures to say that they have epilepsy). Most of these nonepileptic seizures occur in infancy and are associated with high fever arising from infection—thus the term *febrile seizures of infancy*. This type of seizure is rather like the one Clint suffered, with convulsions affecting all four limbs. Febrile seizures occur because the immature infant brain has a lower threshold for seizures than that of an adult.

More than two million Americans have epilepsy. The associated annual health care cost is over $12.5 billion, of which more than 85 percent is related to lost earnings and productivity. Medications make up only about 5 percent of the total costs. These are the cold facts about epilepsy, but they do not capture the enormous social and personal burden that epilepsy places on patients and their families.

## What causes seizures?

Of great interest to me as a neurologist—and to the patient who suffers from epilepsy—is the question of what causes the electrical brain storm that we call a seizure. To understand a seizure, you need to know something about the electrical function of the brain.

The brain is comprised of about 100 billion neurons, each of which is like a little electrically charged battery. At rest, the neuron cell membrane is electrically charged to a potential of about -70 millivolts (mV), which is tiny when compared with the 1.5-volt potential of a double-A battery or the 12-volt battery of a car. When a neuron fires it is a little like a spark between cables attached to the terminals of the car battery. The membrane of the neuron "shorts" out (the technical term is that it depolarizes), and the potential goes from -70 mV to about +20 mV. The action potential—that is, the wave of electricity that spreads along the membrane of the neuron—passes down to the end of the axon. There, at the synapse with the next neuron, the nerve action potential releases a chemical, the neurotransmitter, which diffuses rapidly across the extremely narrow gap between the axon tip and the next neuron.

The neurotransmitter released into the synaptic gap binds to a complex series of proteins called receptors, which are embedded in the cell membrane of the next neuron. This stimulates the next neuron to change its resting membrane potential. That is not to say the second neuron will necessarily fire. While some neurotransmitter receptors are excitatory, causing the second neuron to fire off an action potential down its own axon, other neurotransmitter receptors are inhibitory—that is, they increase the negative resting membrane potential of the second neuron, thus decreasing the likelihood of its firing.

The membrane potential and action potential of neurons result from the movement of atomic particles called ions—principally sodium, potassium, and calcium—through special channels in the nerve cell membrane. We call these ion channels. A special pump, the sodium-potassium pump, exports sodium ions from inside the neuron into the tissue fluid bathing the cell, thereby restoring the resting membrane potential of -70 mV after the action potential has passed.

Neurons send out axons and other branches called dendrites to make synapses with many other neurons of the brain. There are about 60 trillion synapses in the brain. Although everything doesn't necessarily connect to everything else, this interconnected "wiring" of the neurons provides the circuitry through which excitation can spread to all neurons of the brain during a seizure. In the normal brain a global spread of excitation does not occur because inhibitory mechanisms limit the spread.

The brain of a person who suffers from epilepsy differs from that of someone who does not. Patients develop seizures because of an abnormality of their brain. This may be a tumor or scar irritating the adjacent neurons, causing them to fire in an uncontrolled fashion (they are said to have focal epilepsy due to a seizure focus). On the other hand, in patients with what may be called generalized epilepsy, the epileptic brain is more vulnerable to the global spread of excitation. This may result from alterations in ion channels, alterations in the synthesis and release of neurotransmitters, or alterations in the neurotransmitter receptors. Some patients with epilepsy appear to develop this tendency out of the blue with no known reason. Others have a family history and are said to have familial epilepsy. Members of these families must have a mutation of one of the genes related to ion channels, neurotransmitters, or neurotransmitter receptors.

In a sort of vicious cycle, repeated epileptic seizures seem to produce yet more seizures. This is why we neurologists try to keep patients from having repeated attacks. If a seizure focus on one side of the brain continues firing for too long, the neurons on the opposite side of the brain that connect to the epileptic area become epileptogenic themselves. This so-called mirror focus can then cause epileptic seizures in its own right.

Another process that worsens epilepsy following repeated seizures results from damage to the neurons of the hippocampus, in the inner part of the temporal lobes. Every grand mal seizure, like the one Clint experienced, tends to reduce the supply of oxygen to the brain. When Clint's parents first found him, he was stiff and blue in the face because all his muscles were contracted, making it impossible for him to breathe. This is called the tonic phase of the seizure. Clint soon started jerking all over, which is called the clonic phase of the seizure. Neurons of the hippocampus are very sensitive to lack of oxygen, and every seizure causes death of a few hippocampal neurons. The associated hippocampal scarring, called medial temporal sclerosis, can be seen on MRI scans. This scarring can cause epileptic discharges and a vicious cycle of yet more epileptic attacks.

What happens in the brain during a seizure can be likened to a thunderstorm with lightning flashing between the clouds and down to the earth. In the electrical brain storm that we call a seizure, the neurons of the cerebral cortex discharge independently, with no voluntary action on the part of the patient. If the electrical discharge of the neurons spreads to the whole brain, then the person becomes unconscious, and discharges of all the cerebral motor neurons make the muscles of the body jerk violently. A major seizure like Clint's is terrifying to witness and horrible to suffer.

If the electrical discharge remains localized, or focal, to one part of the brain, the person usually remains awake but may have involuntary jerking of one hand, for instance, if the focal seizure affects the motor neurons of the hand area of the cerebral cortex on the opposite side.

If a person has many seizures in his lifetime, then he is said to have epilepsy. People with epilepsy are essentially no different from the rest of us. In fact, anyone can have a seizure if he is exposed to sufficiently strong stimuli. The only difference between someone with epilepsy and someone without it is the epileptic's sensitivity to things that excite their cerebral cortical neurons.

The clearest demonstration of the human vulnerability to seizure is electroconvulsive therapy (ECT). During this therapy, which is still used to treat severe depression that does not respond to medications, electrodes are placed on the scalp and an alternating electrical voltage is applied. When enough voltage is applied to the brain, *any* patient will have a seizure (unless he is under general anesthesia and is paralyzed).

Some individuals suffer seizures as a result of seemingly innocuous stimuli, such as sleep deprivation or too much caffeine. Others have recurrent seizures spontaneously, without any obvious stimulus; they are said to have idiopathic epilepsy, meaning that we do not know what causes it. Yet other patients suffer seizures when something irritates a part of the cerebral cortex. Patients with such an epileptic focus are said to have secondary epilepsy, because the seizures are secondary to some primary cause.

## Tests Used to Diagnose Epilepsy

The first "test" that a doctor needs to conduct when he sees a patient with a presumed seizure is to take a good history. This helps the doctor make sure that it really was a seizure and not something else that looked similar. Someone who faints is often thought to have had a seizure because he falls to the ground unconscious and his limbs may have twitched. However, when we ask such a patient if he had any warning of the attack, he will remember the roaring in his ears, the light-headed feeling, and his vision going dark before he passed out. All these signs are characteristic of a faint. Someone who suffers a seizure generally gets no warning. In Clint's case, there was no doubt that he had had a seizure.

## The EEG

The EEG that I arranged for Clint was performed by a technician, who glued dozens of little disc electrodes to Clint's scalp and connected them to a computer with a skein of wires. In the old days, an EEG machine had dozens of little ink pens that drew squiggles on a wide sheet of paper. Nowadays, EEG machines are paperless. They store all the information on a DVD for the neurologist to review on a large computer monitor. The technician had Clint lie on a bed, first with his eyes open and then with his eyes closed, while the EEG machine recorded Clint's brain waves. Later, he put a bright flickering light in front of Clint's eyes to see if it would induce a seizure. Finally, he continued recording the brain waves while Clint rested on the bed and drifted off to sleep.

The EEG machine was derived from the electrocardiograph (EKG) machine, which is used for recording a person's heartbeat. The pulsing heart works via electrical activity and produces a very characteristic pattern of electrical waves that can be recorded from the chest and limbs. The electrical pulses, called potentials, produced by the brain are much smaller than those produced by the heart. They are also much more complex and less well understood. Nevertheless, potentials can be used to identify epilepsy and many other diseases affecting the brain.

When a neuron fires a nerve impulse down its axon, the passage of that action potential produces a tiny electromagnetic pulse. The total activity of many millions of neurons in an area of the brain produces potentials large enough to be recorded by an EEG machine. When a patient's eyes are open and looking at something, the enormously complex activity of the brain produces a low-voltage EEG that is not very revealing. However, when the patient closes his eyes and relaxes, a waveform called the alpha rhythm normally builds up over the cerebral cortex of the brain at a frequency of about nine cycles per second. The alpha waves probably result from some electrical generator deep in the brain "ticking over" like a car idling, waiting for the eyes to be open so the brain can "step on the gas" and start paying attention to what it sees.

Some of the other "brain waves" recorded on an EEG machine are slower or faster than the alpha rhythm. If the patient is anxious or has taken stimulants, the brain waves have an increased frequency and are called beta waves. When the patient becomes drowsy and goes to sleep, the frequency of the brain waves slows and their amplitude increases; these waves are called theta and delta waves. If a tumor or abscess in a focal area of the brain caused a seizure, the EEG electrodes will record abnormal theta and delta waves around that area. If an area of the brain has been destroyed by a stroke, the EEG will show no electrical activity in that area.

We use EEGs to look for evidence of seizure activity. If a patient has a seizure while linked up to the EEG machine, it produces high-voltage discharges that are unmistakable. If it is possible to determine where in the brain these discharges first appeared before they spread through the whole brain, then this location, which we call the seizure focus, is likely to contain the cause of the seizure. However, seizures rarely occur during EEG recording, and usually all that we can find are a few sharp waves, sometimes followed by a slower wave, that indicate an area of neurons that are abnormally irritable. These series are called spike and wave discharges.

To try to bring out epileptic electrical changes, we sometimes deliberately stress the patient through sleep deprivation, stimulant drugs, or photostimulation with a pulsing light such as the one used in Clint's study. All of these stimuli can induce seizure activity in the brains of susceptible individuals.

The EEG is an old and somewhat limited tool for investigating both normal and abnormal brain activity. Brain waves recorded by an EEG machine are many orders of complexity removed from the brain's individual neurons, as well as the abnormal ion channels and neurotransmitter receptors that are responsible for a seizure. The EEG usually cannot tell us what is causing the epilepsy, and it does relatively little to help us find the seizure focus. Clint's EEG showed only a few spikes and waves on both sides of the brain. I expected to see this pattern, which is associated with idiopathic epilepsy, since I thought it most likely that Clint had a familial tendency toward epilepsy rather than a tumor or abscess in the brain.

## The MRI

Clint's MRI scan came back normal. I collected the CD of the images and reviewed them on my computer. I also reviewed them with my neuroradiologist colleague. I particularly wanted to know if we could see subtle congenital developmental abnormalities of the cerebral cortex that may cause seizures in people of Clint's age. Everything looked normal. It was even more likely that Clint had idiopathic epilepsy.

## Other tests of brain function

Additional tests are occasionally used to study patients with seizures. We can obtain a great deal of information by simultaneously recording the EEG and taking videos of the patient's activities before and during a seizure. Because seizures occur relatively infrequently, video EEG recordings often require admitting patients to the hospital for several days, during which time their antiepilepsy medication is stopped. This may allow one or more seizures to occur and to be captured on the simultaneous video and EEG.

Video EEG recording is used to separate true seizures from so-called psychogenic or pseudo-seizures (I will say more about these later). It can also be used to determine which area of the brain is the first to show an EEG abnormality at the very beginning of a seizure. A less effective but cheaper alternative is an ambulatory EEG. In this test, the patient wears EEG electrodes glued on his scalp and a miniature portable EEG recording machine for two days, while carrying on his normal activities outside the hospital.

Another test available in a few specialized centers is magnetoencephalography. This recording instrument makes use of magnetic waves that can identify the seizure focus in three dimensions more effectively than an EEG machine can. The instrument can detect the electromagnetic wave produced by the electrical pulse of a group of neurons' action potentials.

Yet another test is the positron emission tomography (PET) scanner. This instrument uses radioactive oxygen to show where neurons are consuming more oxygen than in the normal surrounding brain because they are overactive during seizure activity. Often the PET scan shows that a seizure focus is underactive when the patient is not having a seizure. The PET scan can also be used to find a tumor.

Functional magnetic resonance imaging (fMRI) uses the ability of the MRI machine to detect local blood flow. If an area of neurons is overactive or underactive as a result of its being a seizure focus, the fMRI scan can detect an altered local blood flow in that area.

# Clinical Features of Epilepsy

There are many classifications of epilepsy. The World Health Organization, as well as a nongovernmental organization called the International League Against Epilepsy, revise the classifications frequently. This can be very confusing to someone who does not specialize in epilepsy. The most important thing to understand about the various classifications is that seizures can be described in several dimensions, and therefore several different terms may be applied to the same seizure.

## Types of Seizures

Seizures may be *convulsive* or *non-convulsive*, depending upon whether the patient has major abnormal movements during the seizure, like those experienced by Clint. Seizures can be *generalized*, affecting the whole body symmetrically at the same time, or *focal*, starting in one part of the body and usually caused by an abnormality in a particular place in the opposite side of the brain. Seizures can be *symptomatic*, or caused by an underlying injury, such as a brain tumor or an infection like an abscess or encephalitis. If no underlying cause can be found for the seizures, they are called *cryptogenic* or *idiopathic*.

The generalized epilepsies can be broadly separated into *tonic-clonic* or *grand mal seizures*, which were Clint's type of attacks, or *absence* or *petit mal seizures*, in which there is no significant convulsive attack. The term *tonic-clonic* refers to the fact that the limbs alternately go rigid, during the tonic phase, and then jerk back and forth violently, during the clonic phase. The term *absence* refers to the fact that the patient is out of contact with the world, or "absent," during the time of the attack; he is unaware of his surroundings and incapable of responding to questions.

Other, less common, types of seizures include those associated with sudden jerks of the limbs (*myoclonic seizures*) and those in which the patient suddenly drops to the ground and is briefly unconscious but still (*akinetic* or *atonic seizures*, also called drop attacks).

The International League Against Epilepsy currently divides the epilepsies into two categories. *Partial seizures* are like focal epilepsy, though not necessarily relating to a structural abnormality. *Generalized seizures* arise in both cerebral hemispheres and can be either convulsive or nonconvulsive. Partial seizures are further classified as *simple partial seizures*, in which the patient remains conscious, or *complex partial seizures*, in which of the patient's consciousness is impaired at some point during the seizure. Partial seizures may develop all the features of generalized seizures, at which point they are called *secondarily generalized epilepsy*.

## Grand mal seizures

The type of seizure that Clint had is called a tonic-clonic or grand mal seizure. Without warning the patient stops, lets out a cry, and collapses unconscious. Within a few seconds the arms and legs go rigid, the eyes roll upward, and the head is drawn back. The patient takes a breath and then holds it. His face becomes red and then blue due to lack of oxygen. The patient may begin to make strangled noises and often wets himself.

The tonic phase then passes, and the clonic phase begins. All four of the patient's limbs jerk violently, which can result in broken bones, a dislocated shoulder, or a head injury. Violent chewing movements may result in biting of the tongue and cheeks. People trying to help should not put a pencil or spoon between the jaws of someone seizing because this often results in damage to the teeth.

After some time, the clonic convulsion ceases and the patient becomes quiet, though breathing heavily. Usually the tonic-clonic phase lasts three to five minutes. However, repeated seizures may go on for twenty minutes or more. This condition is called status epilepticus. The patient may remain unconscious for ten to fifteen minutes and then wake up feeling confused and slow of thought. He will probably have a good deal of pain in his arms, legs, and back because his muscles were overworked severely during the seizure. His mental state may not return to normal for several hours after the seizure.

The frequency of grand mal attacks varies greatly. Some patients have a dozen attacks a week, while others have an attack once every ten years. The frequency presumably indicates the degree of "irritability" of the brain.

Seizures often occur completely without warning. Patients with epilepsy live with a sword of Damocles hanging over their heads while they wait for the next seizure to strike them down. Sometimes seizures do have direct causes, however. These include stress, sleep deprivation, and excessive caffeine or other stimulants. Patients with epilepsy should avoid these stresses.

Occasionally, an external event can precipitate what is called reflex epilepsy. There was a patient in England whose seizures always happened at the same time each day. His neurologist discovered that the seizure occurred when a BBC radio program played church bells as interval music between programs. The sound of the church bells was inducing the patient to have a seizure. This phenomenon is called musicogenic epilepsy.

Grand mal seizures occur most frequently at night. Sometimes the only evidence of the seizure is that the patient finds on awakening that he has wet the bed.

## Epilepsy and driving

Patients often receive no warning before the onset of a seizure. This makes it dangerous for them to drive a motor vehicle, operate dangerous machines, work at heights, or go swimming without friends who are trained in rescue and resuscitation techniques. These guidelines are important for the safety of both the patient and people around him.

The laws that regulate licensing drivers with epilepsy vary from country to country and from state to state. The common principle is that patients with uncontrolled epileptic attacks should not drive. In some countries, the doctor making a diagnosis of new onset epilepsy is required to provide the motor vehicle licensing authority with the name and demographic features of the patient, who then has his driver's license revoked. The laws generally allow patients to regain their licenses when they can affirm that they are taking antiepileptic drugs and that they have been seizure-free for a certain period of time, usually six months to two years.

Patients can suffer injury and even death during a grand mal seizure. Head injuries, as well as the cumulative effect of oxygen deprivation due to many seizures, can add to the damage. Chronic uncontrolled seizures can impair memory and intellect, collectively called higher cognitive functions. In addition antiepileptic medications have significant side effects. Many of the medications have a sedative effect, and some can produce neurological problems such as cerebellar degeneration, which causes unsteady gait; ataxia (slurred speech); and peripheral nerve damage, termed peripheral neuropathy.

## Familial epilepsy

Epilepsy is sometimes familial, either on its own or hand in hand with certain degenerative diseases. Myoclonic epilepsy often runs in families. While some forms of infantile and juvenile myoclonic epilepsy are benign, others may lead to progressive deterioration of the patient's mental capacity. One fatal form of familial myoclonic epilepsy is called

Lafora's disease. This condition was named after early twentieth-century Spanish neurologist Gonzalo Lafora, who first recognized characteristic abnormal particles in the neurons of these families when he looked at their brains with a microscope. In rare cases, epileptic seizures may also develop in patients with Alzheimer's disease and other neurological degenerations of old age.

## Status epilepticus

Grand mal seizures are usually self-limited and only a few minutes in duration. Attacks can, however, occur in flurries, and occasionally the patient does not wake up between one seizure and the next. If seizures continue for more than twenty minutes, the condition is called status epilepticus. This can be very damaging to the brain due to oxygen deprivation in the face of severe overactivity of the neurons.

In the past, status epilepticus was usually fatal, but with modern medications and intensive care, death is now less common. Treatment involves putting an airway down the back of the patient's throat to provide oxygen to the lungs and blood. After a fast ambulance ride to the nearest hospital, the patient will receive intravenous antiepileptic medications to dampen the seizure activity in his brain. If the medications are unsuccessful, the patient will be placed on artificial ventilation, and he will be given paralyzing drugs to prevent the seizures from affecting his body.

## Petit mal or absence seizures

Petit mal attacks typically occur in children. This is one of the types of partial epilepsy.

A nine-year-old girl named Jennifer was brought to me because her school performance was deteriorating. She was normally an accomplished student, but teachers reported that she had begun daydreaming in class. Jennifer could not explain why she was not doing as well at school. During our first consultation, I was lucky enough to see one of Jennifer's "daydreams." She suddenly stopped talking, stared into space, and began smacking her lips and nodding her head. After five or ten seconds, she came out of the attack and continued with the conversation as though there had been no interruption. I asked Jennifer if she knew that she had had an attack, and she denied that anything had happened.

Absence seizures can come a hundred or more times a day. During the seizure the patient is completely unaware of her surroundings and does not respond to questions or commands. It is therefore not surprising that Jennifer's grades had been dropping. She was "daydreaming" for many minutes each lesson and missed much of what the teacher was saying. I put her on ethosuximide (Zarontin®). Jennifer's attacks stopped, and her school performance improved dramatically.

## Epileptic automatism

Our brains are capable of independent coordinated motor activity of which we are completely unaware. Sleepwalking is the most familiar example. When my oldest son was a child, we would sometimes find him wandering around the house at night. When my wife or I asked him what he was doing, he would mumble some nonsense. We would get him back to bed, and when we talked to him about it the next morning, he had no memory of the episode. Sleepwalking is not epileptic in nature. Rather, it is an aberration of normal sleep that is fairly common in children.

Similar automatic behavior may take place as part of a complex partial seizure, however, and the patient retains no memory of the event. The automatisms are usually simple—the patient may pick at her clothes or mumble—but can at times be complex. I have seen some patients who let out peals of laughter whenever they had a seizure (gelastic epilepsy, from the Greek *gelos* for "laughter") and others who had bouts of uncontrolled crying related to a seizure (dacrystic epilepsy, from the Greek word meaning "crying").

In rare cases, patients with temporal lobe and frontal lobe epilepsies can have rage outbursts or perform actions that are quite out of character as a result of an epileptic discharge. For this reason, epilepsy is sometimes advanced as a defense in murder trials. Since it is impossible to prove or disprove that the accused truly was having an epileptic attack when he committed the murder, most courts have ruled that epilepsy is not a valid murder defense.

## Focal seizures

Patients may have seizures originating in a particular part of the brain. Usually such focal seizures are the symptomatic form of epilepsy. They are caused by abnormalities—which we doctors call lesions—of the brain. The lesions cause focal seizures by irritating nearby neurons of the cerebral cortex so that they produce epileptic discharges. Often, the seizures spread to both sides of the brain to produce secondary generalized epilepsy.

Some focal seizures result from developmental lesions that a patient was born with, such as cysts, malformations of areas of the brain that are abnormal in structure, and abnormal tangles of blood vessels called arteriovenous malformations. Focal epilepsy due to these congenital lesions often begins in childhood.

Some patients with frequent seizures have port-wine stains on their faces. These stains are signs of Sturge-Weber syndrome. The marks are caused by a collection of abnormal blood vessels in the skin of the face. These often are associated with a similar collection of abnormal blood vessels on the brain, which cause epileptic discharges of neurons in that area.

Other causes of focal seizures are brain lesions acquired later in life, such as tumors, abscesses, strokes, head injuries, and encephalitis. Someone who has suffered a major stroke affecting the cerebral cortex has a 50 percent chance of having a seizure in the next ten years. A scar in the brain acts as an irritative focus. One-quarter of patients with a penetrating injury of the brain, such as a bullet wound, develop epilepsy at some point. Rasmussen's encephalitis is a focal inflammatory disease of the brain that gives rise to focal epilepsy in children. This condition is now believed to result from an autoimmune process in which the body produces antibodies against its own brain tissue. Anti-inflammatory treatment and surgical removal of the affected area can sometimes cure Rasmussen's encephalitis.

## Epileptic auras

Many epilepsy patients experience an abnormal neurological manifestation called an aura. The aura tells them they are going to have an attack, sometimes within the next few minutes. A seizure focus in one area of the cerebral cortex may produce epileptic phenomena specific to the normal function of that particular area. For instance, in epilepsy affecting the temporal lobe, where neurons process sensory information, patients often have an aura of sudden fear, taste, or smell. They may also experience a gastrointestinal symptom such as rumbling of the stomach or sudden hunger. Epileptic attacks coming from the medial temporal area, which plays an important part in memory, may result in an aura of a sudden sense of déjà vu—the feeling of having seen or done something before—or a sudden sense of complete confusion, called jamais vu. Because the neurons for hearing are located in the superior temporal lobe, patients with seizures originating in this area may have an aura of specific sounds or a certain piece of music.

An aura associated with generalized siezures may simply be a feeling of restlessness or dread. This sensation might flow from a heightened awareness of everything going on in the brain due to decreased inhibition of the cortical neurons. (Decreased inhibition leads to increased sensitivity to incoming sensory messages and enhanced awareness of spontaneous thoughts.) Many patients report feeling anxious at these times.

*Epileptic march*

John Hughlings Jackson, an English neurologist, was the first to describe the unique focal motor-convulsion pattern that has come to be called the Jacksonian epileptic march. Jacksonian convulsions usually begin with uncontrolled twitching in the thumb or corner of the mouth on the side opposite the lesion in the motor cortex. The twitching may spread to the whole arm and face on that side, and from there may spread to produce a tonic-clonic seizure of both sides of the body. Patients with Jacksonian epilepsy can sometimes stop the attack by grabbing the affected arm. An inexperienced doctor can misinterpret this as indicating that the seizure is not truly epileptic.

A sensory Jacksonian march involves tingling instead of twitching if the epileptic focus is in the sensory area of the cerebral cortex, rather than the motor area. Seizure foci in the occipital lobes are less common. These patients may have auras of flashing lights or more complex visual images in the visual field opposite the lobe of the seizure focus.

# Treatment and Prognosis of Epilepsy

In order to investigate the causes and treatment of epilepsy, researchers have needed to study animals with epilepsy. Some animals, including particular strains of laboratory rats, have spontaneous seizures. A few of the genes responsible for familial epilepsy have been put into mice. These so-called transgenic mice are being used to investigate the basis of familial epilepsy. Focal and secondary generalized epileptic seizures can be induced in laboratory rats via the injection of irritating chemicals, such as penicillin, into the cerebral cortex. Researchers have used these animal models to develop the drugs that we now use to treat patients with seizures.

## Medical treatment

Drug treatment of epilepsy began with the use of bromide and, later, phenobarbital. Both medications are sedatives that decrease the frequency and severity of grand mal epilepsy. In the 1930s, Harvard neurologists Houston Merritt and Tracy Putnam discovered that phenytoin (Dilantin®) is useful for controlling seizures and has a less sedative effect. Since that time, many drugs have been developed for the treatment of seizures. These include ethosuximide (Zarontin®), which is particularly useful for petit mal seizures, and carbamazepine (Tegretol®), which works like Dilantin on convulsive epilepsy.

The treatment of epilepsy has become a highly specialized field. The last twenty-five years have seen an outpouring of new drugs that act on different biochemical pathways, neurotransmitters, and forms of epilepsy. Neurologists often measure the level of antiepileptic drugs in the blood to see if the patient is getting the right amount. A neurologist needs not only to know about the different drugs, their doses, and their applications to various types of epilepsy, but also to understand how the drugs are metabolized in the body and how different drugs interact with one another. The latter body of knowledge is called pharmacokinetics.

When taking an antiepileptic drug, a patient must maintain a blood level high enough to control seizures but not so high as to cause toxic side effects. This range of effectiveness is called the therapeutic range. A drug's therapeutic range is determined by trial and error. It should serve as a guideline for the doctor, not a rigid rule of treatment. Some patients' seizures can be controlled by drug blood levels well below what is generally recognized as the lower end of the therapeutic range. Other patients require blood levels well above the upper end of the therapeutic range to control their seizures, and despite this they experience no side effects.

The rule of thumb is to try to achieve seizure control with just one drug. This is called monotherapy. The neurologist administers the drug known to be most effective for the patient's particular type of seizure. Then he slowly increases the dose over a series of frequent clinic visits.

The patient keeps a diary of his seizures, and the neurologist inquires about side effects known to come from the particular drug.

As soon as the seizures stop, the neurologist stops increasing the dosage, regardless of the patient's drug blood level. On the other hand, if the dose needs to be increased to a level that produces intolerable side effects without controlling the seizures, then the doctor will stop the drug—usually by slowly decreasing the dosage—and try another drug. This is the ideal way to treat epilepsy. It is not always completely effective, however, and multidrug therapy, also called polypharmacy, is sometimes necessary.

No drug is free of side effects. At a high dosage, many antiepileptic medications produce symptoms of intoxication similar to those of drunkenness, such as sedation, unsteadiness when walking, and slurred speech. The drugs may slow mental processes, which adds to the problems that epileptic patients have with dangerous machines and driving. Long-term use of antiepileptics may also damage the cerebellum and peripheral nerves.

Women are advised to avoid getting pregnant while taking antiepileptic drugs because all these medications may damage the developing fetus, particularly in the first eight weeks. If it is not possible to stop the medications because the seizures are too frequent or severe without them, then pregnancy should be avoided—or the prospective parents must fully understand and accept the risk.

## Surgical treatment of seizure disorders

If a brain tumor is responsible for a patient's seizures, it should be removed whenever possible. This is necessary not only because the tumor itself may be dangerous, but also because the seizures sometimes disappear as a result. If an abscess is responsible for the seizures, antibiotics are the desired treatment. However, doctors may need to perform a surgical procedure to collect the pus inside the abscess in order to define the organism and the antibiotics to which it is sensitive.

Surgery also plays an important role in the treatment of patients who have been through the gamut of antiepileptic drugs but are still having three or four seizures a week. These patients are said to have refractory or intractable epilepsy. The type of surgery depends upon the cause of the condition. If the seizures are caused by a congenital developmental abnormality, such as an arteriovenous malformation or a mass of abnormal neurons (a neuronal ectopia) in the cortex of the brain, it may be possible to remove the malformation surgically and thus to cure the epilepsy. However, many of these congenital lesions lie close to exquisitely important parts of the brain, such as the speech center in the left frontal lobe. To remove a lesion from such a location would render the patient unable to speak.

A team of neurosurgeons and neurologists is needed to treat uncontrollable seizures that are wrecking a patient's life. If the standard investigations, such as EEG and MRI, indicate that the epileptic focus is in a region of the cerebral cortex that seems safely removable, the team will do electrocorticography. In this procedure, they seek the exact site where the epileptic discharge originates and the exact nature of the brain adjacent to the malformation. They open the skull and place a grid of electrodes over the area that, as seen on the regular EEG, originates the epileptic discharges. Recordings from individual electrodes may show the exact location of the seizure discharge. It is also possible to put little electric currents into each electrode, one at a time, and to determine the specific role of the part of the brain under that particular electrode. For instance, if cortical electrodes show that the seizures come from the left frontal lobe, and if stimulation by electrodes around the focus produces speech arrest, the neurosurgeon will not be able to remove the malformation without producing aphasia.

Neurosurgeons have found that removing certain parts of the brain can decrease seizures in a nonspecific way. The medial part of the temporal lobe and the hippocampus are parts of the brain from which many seizures arise. Temporal lobectomy—removal of the medial temporal lobe—can greatly reduce or even cure intractable epilepsy. However, this surgery can be done on one side only; early surgical experience showed that removal of both medial temporal lobes produces Korsakoff's syndrome, a devastating condition in which a patient is unable to lay down new memories.

Another part of the brain that neurosurgeons can manipulate to reduce epileptic attacks is the corpus callosum, the structure that connects the right and left halves of the brain. Callosotomy, a procedure in which the corpus callosum is cut, may reduce the severity of intractable generalized epilepsy. After callosotomy, it takes sophisticated neuropsychological testing to detect a deficit in patients. In rare cases, however, callosotomy can produce bizarre neurological effects, which I describe in Chapter 1.

Children who suffered a stroke before birth or in infancy may experience paralysis on the side of the body opposite the stroke (hemiparesis or hemiplegia, depending on the severity of the weakness), together with intractable seizures. Even though the damaged hemisphere has little functioning nervous tissue, it is the source of the epileptic discharges. Surgical removal of this scarred cerebral hemisphere, in a procedure called a hemispherectomy, sounds horrendous, but it can virtually cure epilepsy for some patients. As it turns out, removal of the scarred brain does not greatly increase the hemiparesis. Control of seizures is not guaranteed, however. Furthermore, some patients develop chronic oozing of blood from the cavity after hemispherectomy. The iron pigment released from the blood may damage the whole brain and cause a condition called cerebral hemosiderosis, which impairs mental function.

## Brain stimulation

The brain has both excitatory and inhibitory systems. It is possible to stimulate the inhibitory systems, thereby decreasing a person's tendency to develop a seizure. Vagus nerve stimulation is a procedure in which surgeons place electrodes around the vagus nerve in the neck and attach them to a pacemaker implanted underneath the skin of the chest. The stimulation increases inhibition and lowers the frequency of intractable seizures. It is theoretically possible that deep brain stimulation with fine wire electrodes implanted into specific areas of the brain may inhibit seizures, though the results to date have not been very encouraging.

## Prognosis of epilepsy

Patients with epilepsy, as well as their families, want to know is what is likely to happen in the coming months and years. The prognosis of epilepsy partly depends upon the nature of the underlying disease causing the seizures. If the seizure is caused by a malignant brain cancer, then the average survival of the patient may only be three months, due to spread of the tumor rather than the seizures. If the patient happens to have preexisting severe mental retardation, which is a not uncommon association, then treatment of the epilepsy will not alter the underlying mental retardation.

In the case of idiopathic epilepsy appearing in childhood or adolescence, the prognosis varies with the type of disorder and the frequency of the attacks. In absence or petit mal epilepsy, generally the child will grow out of the condition before reaching adulthood. For children with grand mal epilepsy who have only a few seizures per year—and their seizures are relatively easily controlled with medication—the prognosis is good, though many may need to take antiepileptic medications for much of their lives. However, if attacks are frequent and do not respond to medications, the child may be suffering from one of the degenerative epilepsies, like Lafora's disease.

Frequent attacks of grand mal convulsive epilepsy may damage the brain and cause progressive deterioration of higher mental functions and fine motor control. However, many patients have grand mal seizures only rarely, perhaps one every five or ten years, and usually at night. For them the prognosis is excellent.

Nevertheless, seizures are so scary, and their effects on a patient's life are so great, that some patients continue to take an antiepileptic medication for decades without ever having a seizure. They regard this as insurance against a further seizure. Sometimes they are right, as I found out when I persuaded a patient to come off phenytoin after twenty seizure-free years. He had a nocturnal attack two months later. Fortunately, though my pride was hurt, he wasn't; he had no problem other than a wet bed, and he was able to go back on phenytoin and continue to drive.

## Other Sudden Events That May Be Mistaken for Seizures

*Faints (vasovagal or vasodepressor syncope)*

The main condition to be distinguished from epilepsy is a faint, also termed syncope. I have always been an easy fainter and am well aware of the symptoms of a threatened faint. I begin to feel hot, tingly, unwell, and distanced from my surrounding. I often have a feeling of weakness, a roaring in the ears, and a dimming of vision. If I do not react to these symptoms and immediately either sit down with my head between my knees or lie on the floor, I may lose consciousness and fall. These attacks have come at the most embarrassing times, such as when I am giving an important lecture. Easy fainters know that their attacks often result from psychological stress; in some people they occur at the sight of blood or as a result of severe pain.

During a faint, the autonomic nervous system goes into a disaster mode. This neural circuitry is the part of our nervous system that controls the "unconscious" or autonomous functions of the body, such as the digestive system and blood pressure. It is the primitive system for "fight or flight" that produces a severe increase in blood pressure when we get angry.

In a few animal species, the threat of attack provokes a different response, and the animal rolls over and plays dead; this is where we get the phrase "playing possum." The animal version of disaster mode is presumably like a faint. In humans, it produces slowing of the heart rate and expansion of the blood vessels in the legs and gut. This, in turn, results in the blood pressure's dropping below the level needed to pump the blood all the way up to the brain. As a result, the brain "switches off," and the patient becomes unconscious and collapses. In a horizontal position, since the heart slows but does not stop during a faint, the fainter's blood pressure is sufficient to send blood through the brain and restore consciousness. However, if the fainter stands up too fast, he may faint a second time.

## Cardiac syncope

Cardiac syncope produces a picture similar to that of an ordinary faint, but it results from loss of the heart's power of contraction. This can be caused by a heart attack that weakens the heart muscle or an irregularity of the heartbeat that reduces the amount of blood pumped to the brain. Elderly patients may experience cardiac syncope and faint because of the "sick sinus syndrome," in which the heart's natural pacemaker is not working properly and the heartbeat drops to below half of its normal rate. The treatment is to implant an artificial pacemaker, technically called an internal cardiac pacemaker, under the skin of the chest, with wires going to the heart to keep it beating at a normal rate.

On rare occasions, a person with any type of syncope can have a superimposed seizure while unconscious, due to lack of blood to the brain. When I was a resident in training, I saw many such attacks, because at that time we only used external cardiac pacemakers for people with the sick sinus syndrome. These pacemakers were stimulator boxes that sat outside the body and were connected to the heart via wires that ran through catheters placed in the veins. We could not leave these external pacemakers in place indefinitely and therefore had to try to wean patients off the machine. If the patient's heart did not start beating on its own, he would rapidly become unconscious, and half the patients who lost consciousness would have a tonic-clonic seizure. Ever since those days I have been aware that syncope can cause a convulsion, and therefore that a seizure, particularly in the elderly, can have a cardiac cause.

The worst thing to do for a person who has fainted is to sit him up. I have seen severe brain damage in a person who had a cardiac syncope and was rushed by well-meaning relatives to the hospital while sitting up in the car seat.

Many patients, both young and old, are prescribed antiepileptic drugs because a doctor thought an unconscious spell was an epileptic seizure, when in fact it was syncope. Such a misdiagnosis can cause one of two problems, neither trivial. First, the patient may die if he is not treated correctly for cardiac syncope. Second, if the cause was a simple faint, the patient may commit to taking antiepileptic drugs for years, until an astute physician makes the correct diagnosis.

## Excessive startle

We are all aware that some people startle easily if you come up behind them and make them jump. Rare people have excessive startle reactions due to a condition that goes by the difficult-to-pronounce Greek name of hyperekplexia. This condition may result from a gene mutation of the glycine receptor, one of the inhibitory neurotransmitter receptors. People from several parts of the world have published reports about excessive reactions to being startled. One of these reports, from the late nineteenth century, describes the Jumping Frenchmen of Maine— French-Canadian lumberjacks who most likely inherited this condition. When startled, they would jump around and hit the person who had frightened them.

## Paroxysmal kinesigenic epilepsy

Though the word *epilepsy* is sometimes applied to the rare and fascinating condition of paroxysmal kinesigenic epilepsy, it is better termed *paroxysmal kinesigenic dyskinesia*. This condition features attacks of involuntary movement triggered by sudden (voluntary) movement. I will discuss it more in the chapter on Parkinson's disease and other movement disorders.

## Pseudo-seizures or psychogenic seizures

It is easy to fake a seizure if you have ever seen a true tonic-clonic seizure. Someone might simulate seizures to win a big insurance settlement for a mild bang on the head. This act is called malingering; the attacks are called factitious seizures and they may be different from the pseudo-seizures that I will describe shortly. I have seen many such patients over the years. One was a forty-five-year-old man sent to me by his attorney with a note saying that he had been having seizures since hitting his head at work. While he was telling me his story, he had one of his attacks. He suddenly bent forward, slowly fell to the floor, and flailed his arms and legs around. This went on for ten minutes, during which he neither wet himself nor bit his tongue. Then he "came to," got back on the chair, and continued to tell me in great detail about the mild head injury that he had suffered at work. The picture was so unlike a typical grand mal seizure that I had to conclude that it was a factitious seizure. The attorney was, however, able to convince a jury that the man had developed epilepsy as a result of the head injury, and he won a big settlement. I heard that the attacks disappeared soon after he received the money.

Pseudo-seizures often look very like the attack in the patient I just described. The patient does not injure or wet himself and, when the attack stops, he is immediately able to converse normally, with none of the confusion that characterizes a true grand mal seizure. Experienced neurologists specializing in epilepsy often diagnose pseudo-seizures because the patient has a normal EEG during the attack. In addition, the character of the attacks differs from that of a typical tonic-clonic seizure. When psychologists treat individuals who have pseudo-seizures, they often find that the patients had significant childhood trauma—particularly sexual abuse—or are currently under severe stress.

The real question is whether the patient is consciously producing a factitious seizure, or whether the pseudo-seizures has a psychological (an involuntary or subconscious) cause. Many of these attacks look very similar from one patient to another. Physicians are sometimes too ready to leap to a diagnosis of "hysteria," an old name now replaced by the term *conversion reaction*, meaning that a mental conflict has converted to a bodily form. I believe that the jury is still out with regard to some pseudo-seizures; they lie in the hinterland between psychiatry and neurology. Patients with pseudo-seizures deserve more than simply being told, "Please go away and do not bother me again." At the least they warrant psychological counseling and therapy, particularly until we understand these conditions better.

## Chapter 5

# Multiple Sclerosis

When most people think of multiple sclerosis (MS), they think of a progressive, crippling disease leading to life in a wheelchair within two years and death within five years. This is simply not true for the majority of patients; MS can be remarkably benign for many. Patients who are told they might have MS need to have a clear idea of what this disease is, what it can do, and how we can treat it.

Jean was an intelligent twenty-nine-year-old accountant who came to see me fifteen years ago. She told me she had noticed something wrong with her left leg about three weeks earlier, and it was getting worse. When I asked her to tell me more about what "something wrong" meant, she said she had found herself limping on her left leg and that it had felt tingly. I inquired if she had ever experienced anything else like this, such as a balance problem, weakness or numbness anywhere else, or a problem with vision. She said, "Well, it's funny you should ask. About three years ago, I had some blurred vision. When I tried covering one eye and then the other, I found that only my right eye seemed to be a problem. I thought it must have been an infection, because my eye was a little sore. Anyway, it cleared up in a few weeks."

As Jean walked into my examination room, I saw that she was swinging her left leg. The left leg was a little weaker than the right, and it was slightly stiff when I tried to bend and straighten her knee. This stiffness is what we call spasticity.

Jean's tendon reflexes, which I tested by tapping her knees (patella tendons) with a little rubber hammer, were abnormally brisk on both sides—that is, they jumped more than they should have. To test sensation, I asked her to close her eyes and touched her left leg with a wisp of cotton. She did not feel it. When I tried on the right leg, however, she picked up the touch right away. When I gave her a slight prick with a pin, she told me it felt blunt on the right leg but very sharp on the left. It might seem wrong that pinprick sensation should be reduced on the right leg, while it was the left leg that was spastic and numb to light touch, but this is correct and explained by the way the nerve fiber tracts run in the spinal cord. I checked the strength, reflexes, and sensation in her arms, and everything seemed normal. All this indicated to me that she had a plaque of demyelination on the left side of the spinal cord somewhere in the thoracic region.

I then looked in Jean's eyes with an ophthalmoscope, which helped me see the back of the eye. I was looking for her optic disc, the place where the optic nerve and the arteries and veins for the retina come into the back of the eye. The optic nerve carries the messages for vision from the retina to the brain. In Jean's left eye, the disc had a normal, pink appearance. On the right, however, the disc was much whiter. To a neurologist, this means that some of the nerve fibers in the optic nerve were damaged some time in the past by a patch of inflammation, called an attack of optic neuritis. This must have been the cause of Jean's blurred vision three years earlier.

When I finished the examination, we walked back to my office. Jean looked a little teary. She already suspected what I now considered most probable: she had MS. I said, "We need some more tests, but I want to let you know that one of the things that I am thinking might cause your problem is MS." Through her tears, Jean said, "I was afraid you would say that. I looked up my symptoms, and that's what I came up with."

# What Is Multiple Sclerosis (MS)?

MS was first described by Jean-Martin Charcot (1825–1893) at Hôpital de la Salpêtrière in Paris. Charcot examined many patients with symptoms that we now recognize as those of MS. When some of these patients died, he performed autopsies and examined their brains. He found that the brains had firm, yellowish patches in the white matter. He called these patches *sclérose en plaques.*

The white matter of the brain is composed of axons ("wires") that connect the gray matter (neurons) of the cerebral cortex to the spinal cord. These axons are covered in myelin ("insulation"), which gives the white matter its color. Myelin, just like insulation on an electrical cord, makes nerve signaling more efficient and faster. Charcot showed that the plaques in his patients' brains had lost their myelin, a phenomenon called demyelination. This is why MS is called a demyelinating disease.

Charcot also recognized that many parts of the brain and spinal cord could be involved in the condition he was studying. Patients might experience a relapse, often followed by partial or complete remission, later followed by relapses in new parts of the nervous system. This pattern of attacks, in which many parts of the nervous system are affected, led to the name *multiple sclerosis.*

MS is an autoimmune disease of the central nervous system. The patient's immune system produces antibodies and a special type of white blood cells called T-lymphocytes, both of which react against the myelin in the brain and spinal cord. This autoimmune process is similar to that of rheumatoid arthritis, in which the body produces antibodies that attack the cartilage of the joints.

We do not know for sure what causes any autoimmune disease, but certainly the person's genetic makeup plays a role. A tendency toward autoimmune diseases often runs in families, and some patients develop more than one of these diseases. Perhaps a virus gets into the body, and the immune system produces antibodies that happen to cross-react with a specific organ. Another possibility is that something goes awry in the complex system of checks and balances that controls the immune system, which then begins to treat one of the body's tissues as if it were a foreign invader.

The autoimmune process in MS starts off with inflammation around the veins in the white matter of the brain and spinal cord. White blood cells (T-cells) in the bloodstream stick to the walls of veins and then pass into the tissue. What makes that happen is not yet known. In the central nervous tissue, T-cells react with myelin and release chemicals called chemokines and lymphokines. These chemicals damage the myelin and the cells that produce myelin, which are called oligodendrocytes. The patient's inflamed vein becomes leaky. It lets in antibodies directed against myelin, and the antibodies do further damage. The myelin is stripped off the axons, which become unable to conduct nerve impulses. The whole area of damaged myelin is called an MS plaque.

The demyelination of axons and resultant blockage of nerve impulses cause the symptoms of MS. If demyelination occurs in the optic nerves, they can no longer convey visual impulses, and the patient loses some or all of the vision in that eye. In other parts of the central nervous system, a demyelinated plaque may produce loss of sensation or paralysis.

The axons running through an MS plaque remain intact initially, but they may be destroyed if the inflammation is very intense. Sclerosis, or hardening of the plaques, results from an increase of scar tissue in the brain (formed by supporting cells called astrocytes)—hence, the *sclerosis* part of MS's name.

Usually after a few weeks or months, the inflammation disappears and some myelin re-forms. This allows the axons to conduct nerve impulses again, leading to partial or complete recovery of function and remission of symptoms—for instance, the recovery of vision in an affected eye. As Charcot discovered, however, another attack of MS may occur somewhere else in the central nervous system at a later time, producing a clinical relapse.

As I will describe later, MS plaques can be seen on MRI scans. Interestingly, many of these plaques cause no symptoms. This is probably because we cannot perceive the activity of large areas of the brain's white matter (we might call these silent areas).

MS is much more frequent than most people realize. When MRI scans became available, they showed that MS is 20 times more frequent than was thought to be the case in Charcot's time. If the diagnosis of MS is defined as a positive MRI *and* the presence of symptoms, the number of people in the United States with MS is quite small—about 60 to 80 per 100,000 people. However, a typical MRI appearance of MS (regardless of whether the patient has symptoms) is seen in about 250 per 100,000 people. This means that about two-thirds of people with a typical MRI appearance of MS never have symptoms of the disease.

In the United States, about three people per 100,000 are diagnosed with MS each year. Nearly 400,000 people—one in 750 Americans—currently live with MS. Many more people have a "touch" of MS, as I will describe later. The total annual cost of treating a patient with established MS is about $50,000, a third of which is for medications. The estimated annual cost of MS in the United States is over $7 billion.

MS has a skewed geographical distribution in the world. Regions populated by people of Northern European stock have the highest frequency of the disease. Progressively less MS occurs in regions populated by non-Europeans. People of Northern European stock have a higher incidence of MS than Africans. Nevertheless, African Americans living in the United States have a higher incidence of MS than people living in the Africa. Living in a region for the first two decades of one's life seems to imprint the geographical risk on people, even if they move to a region of different incidence later in life.

MS has familial tendencies. The general population has a one in 750 chance of contracting the disease. However, the risk increases to one in 40 for parents, children, and siblings of a person with MS. Nevertheless, the genetic basis is not very strong, since the identical twin of a patient with MS has only a 25 percent risk of developing the disease. Put another way, a person's chance of developing MS increases twenty-fold if a parent or sibling has the disease, while it increases two hundred-fold if an identical twin has MS.

First attacks of MS occur most frequently in patients between the ages of sixteen and sixty, with a peak of about age thirty. However, I have seen people as young as three and as old as eighty-four with new-onset MS. Women are affected about twice as frequently as men until the age of about fifty, after which the gender ratio is equal.

## Tests Used to Diagnose MS

The tests used to diagnose MS have become quite reliable in the last decade. Neurologists still need to apply some skill in interpreting them, however.

I arranged for Jean to have blood tests looking for vitamin $B_{12}$ levels, infections such as syphilis and HIV, and autoimmune diseases such as lupus. These tests ensure that the patient's symptoms do not arise from some other condition. However, the finding of a low vitamin $B_{12}$ level or a positive lupus test does not mean that a patient is free of MS; the person may have two separate conditions. But an abnormal blood test should raise the suspicion of a different diagnosis.

I arranged for Jean to have an MRI scan of her brain for two reasons. First, we could rule out strokes and tumors, which could cause symptoms like hers. Second, we could see if multiple abnormal patches had developed in the deep white matter of her brain. Somewhat similar patches are seen in patients with high blood pressure, diabetes, ministrokes, or previous head injuries. A good neurologist will look at the MRI scans to make sure that suspicious patches are of the type and in a location suggesting MS.

Many patients who have an MRI for a common complaint like frequent headaches receive a radiologist's report describing changes that "could be compatible with MS." Patients often come to see me in terror, saying, "They say I have MS. Am I going to be crippled and die?" Most of these patients do not have MS. Instead, they have changes in their brains that occur with age, high blood pressure, diabetes, and many other conditions. These changes look slightly different from the plaques characteristic of MS, and I am able to reassure the patients that they do not have MS. The patients often say, "Doctor, you do not know how much you have done for me today. You have given me my life back." These radiologists' reports keep MS specialists and a few graybeards like me in business.

Back in the old days, when I was in my neurology training, most of the current MS tests were not available. We used X-rays to rule out brain tumors and conducted simple tests of the cerebrospinal fluid, which often carries telltale signs of MS. At that time, we used the hot bath test to add more certainty to an MS diagnosis. Because fever worsens the neurological disabilities of people with MS, we would heat up the patient to see if she developed any new neurological sign that was not present when she had a normal body temperature. It was strange to see a patient, often a young woman, lying in a bathing suit in a steaming hospital bath, with a young doctor checking her visual acuity and doing repeated neurological examinations.

As a young resident I did some research to better understand this phenomenon. I studied a group of patients with MS and another group with other neurological diseases, such as stroke and Friedreich's ataxia. I put a heating frame over the patients and gradually raised their body temperature by two degrees Fahrenheit. This procedure reduced muscle strength by 40 percent in patients with MS but only 10 percent in patients with other neurological diseases. The muscle strength of both groups of patients returned to the preexisting level when their body temperature returned to normal. This experiment showed that axons partly demyelinated by MS lose their ability to conduct nerve impulses when a patient's body temperature rises by only a small amount.

Jean returned to see me a week after the blood tests and MRI were completed. She brought the MRI scan for me to look at. The blood tests were all normal, but the neuroradiologist reported a dozen lesions in the white matter of the brain that might have been caused by MS. I showed Jean the scan and pointed out the patches. I was frank with her: "This is not as good as I hoped. Many people like you have only one or two patches on the MRI, suggesting that they have a benign form of MS. You have a dozen patches, which may mean that the prognosis is not as good as I had hoped. However, we do need to do a spinal tap to confirm that this is MS, and not some other condition."

The cerebrospinal fluid (CSF) is the liquid lying around the brain and spinal cord. It is often abnormal in patients with MS. We can obtain a sample of the CSF by inserting a fine needle into the bottom of the spine while the patient is under local anesthesia. This test is called a spinal tap or lumbar puncture. In MS, signs of inflammation often appear in the CSF. There is an increase in the gamma-globulin content (the component of the CSF that contains antibodies) and the number of white blood cells. The CSF also often contains positive oligoclonal bands, which are distinctive immune system protein formations that confirm a chronic autoimmune process somewhere within the central nervous system. These abnormalities in the CSF do not *prove* that the patient has MS; they sometimes occur in other autoimmune and inflammatory diseases affecting the brain. The neurologist needs to consider the CSF findings together with all the other information before finally diagnosing MS.

Jean had already read about the spinal tap test, and she looked unhappy. I told her all about the procedure and reassured her that it is not as bad as she feared. She came back a week later for me to tell her the results, which confirmed that her CSF had an increased number of white blood cells (especially T-lymphocytes), an increased gamma-globulin content, and positive oligoclonal bands. Taken together, Jean's symptoms, the MRI, and the CSF result confirmed that she had MS.

## Clinical Features of MS

Jean was fairly typical of patients with MS. As I have mentioned, the condition tends to affect people in their twenties and thirties, and women are affected twice as often as men until age fifty. Temporary blurred or lost vision in one eye, due to an attack of optic neuritis, is the first sign of the disease in about one-third of patients. Other MS-related attacks can cause double vision, unsteadiness of walking (ataxia), or weakness or numbness of an arm or leg, depending on where in the central nervous system the MS plaque occurs. If the attack affects the spinal cord, the patient may lose the ability to walk or to feel her legs, and she may lose control of her bladder.

In most patients, the symptoms of the attack develop gradually over a few days, and the loss of neurological function may last for days to months. Eventually, in most patients, the neurological deficit decreases and may even totally disappear. This is called remission. Many patients have one or more subsequent attacks (called relapses) due to new plaques of demyelination, which often develop in a region different from the one that caused the first attack. These are the characteristic clinical features suggesting a diagnosis of MS.

Neurologists have long recognized that some patients with MS appear remarkably unconcerned about their degree of disability. This is akin to *la belle indifférence* that characterizes conversion reaction (formerly termed hysteria). Neurologists believe this lack of concern happens because MS plaques may impair nerve signaling in the frontal lobes, where the capacities to react to stress and to control emotions are localized. Because of this emotional indifference, many patients with MS are initially diagnosed with a psychological disorder. This is unfortunate, as it may lead to the patient no longer trusting the doctor. Dealing with MS requires that the doctor and patient have an excellent working relationship and mutual respect.

We used to advise young women with MS to avoid pregnancy because some studies had suggested that pregnancy increased the risk of relapse. More recent studies, however, have indicated that the chances of relapse are actually reduced *during* pregnancy but increased in the first three months *after* delivery. The latest evidence suggests that attacks of MS may be more frequent for about two years after pregnancy.

Psychological stress can lead to relapse or overall deterioration in all the autoimmune diseases, and this is certainly true for MS. Stress, viral infections, and immunizations may alter the balance between factors enhancing the immune system and those suppressing it, thereby predisposing patients to relapse. Several of my patients have had devastating relapses of MS following a divorce, surgery, or the death of a loved one. It is generally advised that patients with MS avoid immunizations unless they are absolutely essential.

Patients with advanced crippling MS may develop significant cognitive impairment, ranging from poor memory to lack of judgment. In addition, though this is not well recognized by neurologists, cognitive changes can be the only manifestation of the disease, at least at the beginning.

Carolyn was a forty-five-year-old university professor who came to see me because she found herself unable to concentrate or to communicate clearly. For a year she had suffered from severe fatigue. When I examined her, her nervous system seemed perfectly normal, and she did fine on my simple tests of mental function.

Like several neurologists who had examined her before me, I was tempted to conclude that Carolyn's problem was psychological and related to depression. However, I arranged for her to be tested by a neuropsychologist. These tests showed that Carolyn was functioning at an IQ of 120, significantly below her previous level of 160. Now, it is always possible for a patient to falsify her answers on these tests and to appear to be worse than she really is. However, the tests are designed to detect false answers, and experienced neuropsychologists almost always detect them. The tests confirmed that Carolyn had particular problems in the fields of concentration and complex mental tasks.

I arranged a brain MRI, which showed a few questionable lesions in the deep white matter of Carolyn's brain that looked like the plaques seen in MS, though it was not enough evidence to make a diagnosis of MS. Nevertheless, I thought it likely that Carolyn was suffering from MS with an unusual initial symptom of cognitive problems. Over the next few years, she gradually developed a few abnormal neurological signs, and further MRI changes confirmed the diagnosis of MS.

Another patient with isolated cognitive problems was a radiologist who recognized that he was just not as sharp as he had been and worried that he would overlook abnormalities in his work. He sought my help, and his brain MRI showed a few suspicious white-matter lesions. He later developed some abnormal neurological signs of MS.

Both of these patients had to accept permanent disability because of their cognitive problems resulting from MS, though I had to fight with their insurance companies to explain this. We now know that MS can attack oligodendrocytes and the small amount of myelin that lies in the cerebral cortex. High field-strength MRI scanners can now show the demyelinated plaques in the cerebral cortices of patients with MS.

## Treatment and Prognosis of MS

When I told Jean that the tests had confirmed a diagnosis of MS, she said, "This is terrible! How long do I have to live?" I said, "Look, being told you have MS is not great, but the first thing you have to know is that MS is *not* always as bad as you think."

Multiple sclerosis is a relatively common neurological disease. It used to be considered a progressive, paralyzing, and fatal disease. This is because in the decades that followed Charcot, neuropathologists were the only ones able to make the diagnosis—and neuropathologists see only patients who have died. However, as neurologists gradually became able to make the diagnosis in living patients, they realized that many patients lived a normal life span.

In the early 1950s, Scottish neurologist Douglas McAlpine published a number of papers under the title of *Benign MS*, in which he describes patients who appeared to have typical MS, but they had very few attacks and did not become disabled or die. We now know that MS is considerably more benign than early neuropathologists thought. Most patients with MS have a normal life span, and over half suffer no disability. Also, now we have medications that can reduce the frequency of attacks and the progression of neurological disability. Overall, the prognosis of MS is vastly better today than when I first started my career in neurology.

Many years ago, I studied more than seventy patients with optic neuritis, the condition that caused the blurring of Jean's vision three years before I saw her. The patients in my study had been followed for up to twenty years. I found that only 20 percent developed definite MS on clinical grounds. Another 30 percent had some further neurological episodes or signs upon examination but did not develop major disability sufficient to diagnose definite MS. Half the patients had no further neurological problems. Later studies have demonstrated that a positive MRI showing plaques in the brain at the time of the optic neuritis attack suggests that the patient will develop further attacks of MS in the future. If there are no plaques, however, the later development of MS is much less likely.

Up to half of MS patients have the benign form of the disease; they may have one or two attacks and then never have another one. Most people with MS live a normal life with little or no disability. One long-term follow-up study found three-quarters of people still alive thirty years after their MS diagnosis, and more than two-thirds were still working and walking. On average, most of a patient's MS attacks occur in the first five years after diagnosis, and half the attacks are over by the first two years. Jean had already passed through a good deal of the highest-risk period.

After I told Jean about the results of the tests and the causes of MS, her next question was an insightful one: "You said that MS might be due to a virus getting into my nervous system. Can I take an antibiotic to kill the virus?" I replied, "No. Unfortunately, there is no evidence that the virus remains in the body when the MS begins, and we do not have very effective drugs against viruses."

When I first saw Jean, we had corticosteroids (for simplicity, let's call them steroids) for treating an acute attack of MS, anticancer drugs like cyclophosphamide (Cytoxan®), and a newly released drug called beta-interferon (Betaseron®). Forty years before, when cortisone was first discovered, it was shown to be effective for the treatment of autoimmune diseases like rheumatoid arthritis. When it was tried in patients with an attack of MS, it shortened the attack and increased the rate of recovery. However, steroids just bring back function more quickly; they do not make the recovery any more *complete* than it otherwise would have been. Nevertheless, steroid therapy can get a patient walking better or seeing out of a blind eye more rapidly than without this treatment. Steroids can be given as pills by mouth or by injection into a vein. The treatment is usually given for only a few weeks and then stopped.

Jean and I had to decide whether to use steroids for her recent relapse of MS. I shared with her the fact that some neurologists like one treatment, while others like another: "If you put three doctors into a room to decide on the best way to treat a patient, you will get five different opinions." This is certainly the case with regard to steroid treatment. Some neurologists swear by a course of prednisone pills for a relapse of MS. Others think steroids by mouth produce more relapses after the course of treatment has finished, and they prefer to use high-dose intravenous steroids. Jean's walking was already improving, and we decided against using steroids.

After steroids, the next advance in the treatment of MS was the discovery that immune-suppressing drugs used in chemotherapy—such as cyclophosphamide (Cytoxan®), azathioprine (Imuran®), and mitoxantrone (Novantrone®)—can benefit patients with MS. These drugs are relatively toxic, and high doses can result in significant side effects, including nausea, hair loss, and anemia. They are now largely used as drugs of last resort if none of the newer anti-MS drugs are working.

I did recommend to Jean that she take the newly released beta-interferon. I warned her that she would probably feel as though she had a mild attack of the flu for twenty-four hours after each injection. Acetaminophen (Tylenol®) or aspirin can suppress these flu-like symptom. Jean took these beta-interferon injections for the next two years and has never had another attack. The last time I saw her, she was a partner in her firm and had two teenage daughters.

In the fifteen years since I first saw Jean, several new classes of drugs have been shown to suppress MS. Glatiramer (Copaxone®), a drug that was synthesized to resemble myelin basic protein (a component of myelin in the central nervous system), reduces the number of relapses of MS. The beta-interferons (Betaseron®, Avonex®, and Rebif®) reduce the number of relapses and MS plaques.

The latest MS drug, natalizumab (Tysabri®), is an antibody produced by cells in tissue culture. It binds to integrin, a molecule on T-cells that helps them stick to the walls of blood vessels. Natalizumab inhibits T-cells from getting into the brain and thereby prevents relapses of MS. Unfortunately, when beta-inteferon and natalizumab were given to MS patients together, a small number of them developed a different and dangerous type of neurological disease called progressive multifocal leukoencephalopathy (PML). PML is caused by the recurrence of the polyoma virus. We are all exposed to this virus in childhood, and it lies dormant in our bodies after the initial mild infection. If a person's immune system is sufficiently suppressed, the polyoma virus can break out of control and produce this new and potentially lethal infection of the brain. The combination of beta-interferon and natalizumab suppresses the immune system too much, so the drugs are no longer given together.

Not every patient does as well as Jean. Peter was thirty-five years old when I first saw him, and he had developed secondary progressive MS. He had had several relapses in the first two years, and then he had become progressively more disabled. Eventually Peter was unable to walk and incontinent of urine, and he had unsteady arms and slurred speech. He had taken several five-day courses of high-dose intravenous steroid for his early relapses. These produced some improvement, and he had several admissions to a rehabilitation unit that initially helped him to walk with a cane. I treated Peter with baclofen (Lioresal®), which acts against spasticity, or stiffness of the limbs.

Three other drugs can decrease spasticity: diazepam (Valium®), tizanidine (Zanaflex®), and botulinum toxin (Botox®) injections. In my experience, baclofen by mouth causes less drowsiness than diazepam and tizanidine; it can also be put directly into the CSF via a tube passing from an infusion pump implanted below the skin, like a cardiac pacemaker. When put into the CSF in relatively high concentrations, baclofen reduces spinal spasticity without inducing excessive sleepiness. The infusion pump can be programmed via an external magnet to deliver regulated amounts of baclofen at different times of the day. It is refilled at intervals by a needle inserted through the skin into the pump reservoir. A baclofen pump proved remarkably helpful for Peter, and he became able to walk with a walker.

Botulinum toxin, a poison produced by the bacterium that causes the form of food poisoning called botulism, is widely used as a treatment for wrinkles. When injected into stiff, spastic muscles, it may reduce the disability. For someone like Peter, who had severe spasticity of the legs, Botox has to be given with multiple injections into many muscles, which is often impractical.

Rehabilitation can help patients get around the effects of MS. For an acute disabling attack of MS, rehabilitation takes place in a hospital. This often leads to good results. In the United States outpatient rehabilitation is unfortunately limited, particularly because of rules imposed by Medicare and the health insurance companies.

Significantly affected MS patients need the help of many specialists, including neurologists, urologists, rehabilitation specialists, physical and occupational therapists, psychologists, social workers, wheelchair and seating experts, and nutritionists. Ideally, these services would be housed in multidisciplinary clinics that would provide one-stop shopping and be available everywhere in the country. It would be much more convenient for a patient to spend half a day in a multidisciplinary clinic than to have to attend several appointments with different health care providers.

Such clinics are usually only available in MS research centers, which provide other additional benefits. Most neurologists who specialize in MS have seen hundreds or thousands of patients. They know the disease inside and out. They are also often able to involve patients in trials of new drugs that may provide additional relief. Most important, because of their wealth of experience, these specialists can provide the best care possible for all the symptoms of the disease. These include mobility aids such as walkers, wheelchairs, and scooters, as well as braces to hold up the foot of a patient with a foot drop.

Patients with spinal cord MS lesions often have incontinence of urine. This problem can range from urge incontinence, in which the patient is aware of the need to urinate but cannot hold it long enough to get to the bathroom, to total incontinence, when the bladder suddenly empties without warning. Several medications, like oxybutynin (Ditropan®) and tolterodine (Detrol®), can slow the bladder's opening to give the patient more time to get to the bathroom. Devices that can help severely incontinent patients range from condom urinals for males to surgically implanted devices (artificial sphincters) that allow the patient to control when his bladder is emptied.

Sexual dysfunction is a major problem for men with MS because the disease causes erectile dysfunction. Aids that partially restore sexual capacity, if not full orgasm and ejaculation, range from drugs to enhance erectile function—like sildenafil (Viagra®), tadalafil (Cialis®) and vardenafil (Levitra®)—to penile implants. Neurologists often refer patients with erectile dysfunction to urologists for investigation and treatment.

I have had to tell many people that they have MS, and I am only too aware of the shock that the news causes. Not surprisingly, about one-third of patients with MS suffer significant depression at some time during their illness. The professional help of psychologists or psychiatrists, as well as treatment with antidepressant medications such as sertraline (Zoloft®), escitalopram (Lexapro®), and bupropion (Wellbutrin®), are often helpful.

Some patients with MS develop sudden, intense emotional changes and reactions. This causes uncontrollable spasms of crying in response to a mildly sad stimulus, such as talk of a grandmother who died ten years earlier. A few patients experience uncontrollable laughter as well as crying, and the laughter and crying can be paradoxical. One of my patients had to be wheeled out of a relative's funeral because he had burst into peals of uncontrollable laughter. Treatment with antidepressant medications can help patients to gain control of their emotions.

This condition—variously called emotional lability, emotional incontinence, or pseudobulbar affect—results from damage to the brain's frontal lobe connections, which control the lower motor neurons of the bulbar region. This damage produces a condition termed pseudobulbar palsy, which is most common in patients with ALS (Lou Gehrig's disease). The prefix *pseudo* does not imply that the condition is false or that the patient is faking symptoms. It simply means that the condition looks somewhat like the lower motor neuron type of bulbar palsy but is really due to problems at higher levels of the brain.

After about five years of gradual worsening, Peter's condition stabilized. It has remained unchanged for several years. He walks with a tricycle walker for short distances and uses a wheelchair for long trips. His speech is slurred. He can feed himself, though it is a little messy because of the ataxia causing unsteadiness of his hands.

Peter's MS was not the worst that I have seen, but it was certainly not the benign type that affects many patients. There is still some controversy about the prognosis of multiple sclerosis. Many neurologists specializing in MS believe that the disease is eventually progressive, leading to Peter's type of disability. However, private practice neurologists, who tend to be the ones to see patients in the early stages of MS, are impressed by the high proportion of patients who have a relatively benign form and never get referred to an MS research center.

## Other Demyelinating Diseases

The term *demyelinating* means that the insulating material, myelin, surrounding the nerve axons (the "wires" of the brain) is damaged. The demyelinating diseases include disorders that are much rarer than MS. I already mentioned one of them, PML. This disease came about unexpectedly when doctors combined beta-inteferon and natalizumab. PML may also occur in people who have suppressed immune systems, such as patients with AIDS or those receiving immunosuppressive treatment for a kidney or heart transplant.

Other patients have degeneration of the myelin caused not by autoimmune processes but rather by inherited abnormalities of myelin biochemistry. Immune therapy is ineffective for such patients since they do not have an autoimmune disease, and researchers are now looking for ways to correct the biochemical defect. One of these diseases is adrenomyeloleukodystrophy, in which a gene mutation impairs the body's ability to break down very long-chain fatty acids. Treatment with Lorenzo's oil, bone marrow transplantation, and gene therapy are all being tried to treat this condition.

Refsum's disease is another rare disorder of myelin biochemistry that predominantly affects the peripheral nervous system. The patient has an inherited inability to break down phytanic acid—a dietary component derived from chlorophyll, the green pigment of plants—and a resultant disruption of the myelin sheaths. Doctors treat this disease by removing all sources of phytanic acid from the diet or by washing the phytanic acid out of the body with long courses of plasma exchange.

## Chapter 6

# Parkinson's Disease and Other Movement Disorders

Parkinson's disease can conjure up a frightening picture of a stooped old man who is shuffling, drooling, and shaking. People fear Parkinson's disease because they think it is a death sentence preceded by a jail term of being locked in an unresponsive body. While that may have been an accurate picture of the disease some years ago, treatment can now alleviate much of the disability and keep people in good physical condition for years.

Many celebrities have suffered from Parkinson's disease—Michael J. Fox, Muhammad Ali, Janet Reno, and Johnny Cash, to mention just a few. Several celebrities have worked with national organizations devoted to advancing awareness and understanding of the disease. They have all helped make the public aware that someone with Parkinson's can lead a happy and productive life. It is also important to know that many conditions look somewhat like Parkinson's disease but are not. These diseases are grouped together under the term *movement disorders*. I will come back to them after describing typical Parkinson's disease.

Carlos was a fifty-eight-year-old senior captain for one of the major airlines. He told me that his leg had shaken uncontrollably after he had landed his jumbo jet in a typhoon somewhere on the other side of the globe. The wind was coming from 45 degrees left of the runway, and he had to come in with the plane pointing into the wind, with hard right rudder and left aileron, so that the plane would fly straight down the runway. As he touched down he had to straighten out the plane immediately and align it with the runway, then fight the wind until the plane slowed. After he taxied off the active runway he found that his right leg was trembling, and he could not understand why. He said to me, "I love flying, and I'm proud of being able to land under difficult conditions. I was not scared."

I found a slight trace of Parkinson's disease when I examined Carlos. He had little facial expression, and his right arm had a hint of stiffness when I wiggled it. I said, "Well, you are not going to like this, but I think the shaking of your leg was the first sign of Parkinson's disease." Knowing how much pilots like flying, I anticipated his response. He said, "Gee, doc, that's terrible. I was hoping to keep going till they make me retire at sixty. If you tell the FAA medical guys that I have Parkinson's disease, they'll ground me. Can't you do something to keep me flying for another couple of years?"

I told Carlos I would do what I could to keep him flying. I advised him to take medical leave for a month and gave him levodopa (Sinemet®), the standard medication for Parkinson's disease. When he came back to see me four weeks later, I could not detect a trace of Parkinson's disease. I almost wondered if my initial diagnosis had been wrong. At Carlos's request I contacted the Federal Aviation Administration's medical examiner and shared all this information with him. As a result of my discussion with the chief medical officer, Carlos was allowed to keep his airline transport pilot license, as long as he continued the medication and saw me regularly.

A year later, I saw a little tremor in Carlos's right hand and increased his dose of levodopa. Again, this sign of Parkinson's disease disappeared with the added treatment. As required by the airline, Carlos retired at the age of sixty but continued to fly, delivering airplanes around the world. Three years after he first came to see me, and after several more increases in his medication, I found that I could not completely relieve all the signs of the Parkinson's disease. I told Carlos that he would have to give up flying. He fought me on my decision, but I reminded him that flying requires superb reflexes and coordination. When I showed him the slowing of his reaction time, he stopped fighting me.

I went on seeing Carlos for the next six years and adjusted his medications as needed. His walking slowed, and his writing became tiny, which is a common change in patients with Parkinson's disease. He did not develop any of the writhing movements, called dyskinesias, that can complicate the treatment of advanced Parkinson's disease. Carlos continues to enjoy a happy retirement, though he still misses flying.

## What Is Parkinson's Disease?

Sir James Parkinson (1755–1824) was an English physician, paleontologist, and political radical. In 1817 he first described the condition we now call Parkinson's disease in an elegant monograph called *An Essay on the Shaking Palsy*. The next major advance was the recognition that the brains of patients with Parkinson's disease lose the dark staining of the substantia nigra (an area at the front of the midbrain, the upper part of the brain stem). Swedish pharmacologist Arvid Carlsson discovered dopamine in the basal ganglia of the brain in the mid-1950s, and for this he shared the Nobel Prize for Medicine in 2000. Another pharmacologist, Oleh Hornykiewicz of the University of Vienna, showed that the basal ganglia of patients with Parkinson's disease have low levels of dopamine. Although this discovery led to all the medications we now use to treat the disease, Hornykiewicz did not receive the recognition of a Nobel Prize.

More than one million people in the United States have Parkinson's disease. As with Alzheimer's disease and ALS, Parkinson's is more frequent in older populations. In people over the age of seventy, almost one in a hundred has Parkinson's disease.

Patients with Parkinson's disease have several different difficulties with movement. Parkinson's disease is therefore grouped with similar conditions in the category called movement disorders. Parkinson's patients have very slowed movement, marked stiffness, and loss of facial expression. They also often have a spontaneous tremor of the hands. We are now beginning to understand how these two separate abnormalities of movement are produced in patients with Parkinson's disease.

Parkinson's disease results from degeneration of a small group of neurons in the midbrain, which is at the top of the brain stem at the center of the skull. Because these neurons contain a black pigment called melanin, this cluster of cells is called the substantia nigra (Latin for "black substance"). The neurons project their axons to the basal ganglia—paired structures lying just above the midbrain—and release a neurotransmitter called dopamine. Dopamine is the chemical that allows the substantia nigra neurons to control some of the neurons of the basal ganglia. The loss of these connections and this neurotransmitter causes the symptoms of Parkinson's disease. Some neurons in the basal ganglia stimulate others neurons, while others inhibit them. Some feed back onto themselves either to stimulate or to inhibit their own firing of nerve impulses. Some of the neurons fire only when they are stimulated. Others fire continuously in a rhythmic fashion and then stop firing when they receive inhibitory nerve impulses. All these different types of neuron interaction are found in the basal ganglia.

The brain controls movements through the interaction of a series of relay centers. These centers include the motor area of the cerebral cortex, the basal ganglia, the substantia nigra, the cerebellum, and the motor neuron pools in the spinal cord. The relay centers convert the decision to move one leg into the elegant steps of a ballet dancer. The signal to move the leg is magnified and refined as it passes down from center to center, so that messages from a small number of motor cortical neurons reach the many motor neurons in the spinal cord that produce the movements of walking or dancing. Stored in these circuits are the motor memories of various movements—these memories are called motor engrams. With the help of motor engrams, once the movement has been practiced, perfected, and memorized, a relatively simple message from the motor cortex can be translated into the delicately balanced pirouette of the ballerina or a baseball pitcher's fastball.

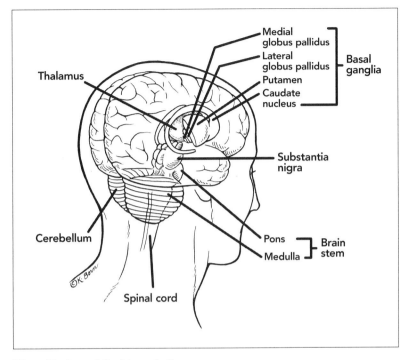

*Fig. 6:* **Brain and Parkinson's disease**
The death of neurons of the substantia nigra impairs the signaling of movement circuits, particularly those of the basal ganglia, leading to the symptoms of Parkinson's disease.

Researchers have found they can tag the receptors for dopamine with a radioactively labeled form of dopamine that lights up the basal ganglia in a healthy person. This procedure is called a positron emission tomography (PET) scan. PET scans of patients with Parkinson's disease show lower than normal activity in the basal ganglia. This demonstrates the loss of dopamine-producing nerve endings coming from the substantia nigra.

Death of substantia nigra neurons removes their connection with the neurons of the basal ganglia. One effect of this is to remove their control over the rhythmically firing neurons, thereby giving rise to a tremor. Death of substantia nigra neurons also takes them out of the circuit that facilitates and speeds up fine movement. This produces slowness of the limbs (neurologists call this bradykinesis) and stiffness (rigidity). It also prevents many of the associated movements that we all do unconsciously, such as standing erect and swinging our arms when we walk, or letting our faces reveal our emotions. Patients with Parkinson's disease therefore are stooped and their arms hang down when they walk. Their faces show very little expression.

## What Causes Parkinson's disease?

In explaining the cause of Parkinson's disease, it is most important to know what makes the neurons of the substantia nigra die. Since Parkinson's disease occurs predominantly in people's senior years, it has been suggested that these neurons age prematurely. However, since we still do not completely understand normal aging, this suggestion does not help us understand Parkinson's disease.

Nevertheless, we have some clues as to what triggers the death of substantia nigra neurons. Five to 10 percent of patients with Parkinson's disease have family members affected by the same condition. Scientists have discovered more than twenty different genes that are mutated in different families with Parkinson's disease; these genes go by such exotic names as alpha-synuclein, parkin, LRRK2, and PINK1. The discovery of genes responsible for familial Parkinson's disease has allowed neuroscientists to introduce the mutated genes into cells in tissue culture and into animals such as the fruit fly and mouse. These so-called transgenic animals have been used to show us how these mutant genes produce proteins that are toxic to neurons and thus cause cell death.

Most cases of Parkinson's disease are sporadic—that is, there is no clear family history, and the disease seems to appear out of the blue. Thus, in most patients, it seems likely that both genetics and environmental factors are involved in causing the disease.

Research into the cause of Parkinson's disease has linked pesticide exposure to an increased risk of the disease. The brains of patients who died of Parkinson's disease have greater amounts of pesticides than the brains of patients who died of other conditions. However, since the disease was recognized well before the advent of the chemical industry, it seems unlikely that we can blame man-made poisons for Parkinson's disease. Toxins that damage the mitochondria (the energy factories of every cell in the body, including neurons) can cause Parkinson's-like changes in animals. Curiously, smokers appear to be somewhat protected against developing Parkinson's disease compared with nonsmokers. However, the dangers of many other smoking-related diseases far outweigh the benefits of preventing Parkinson's disease.

Viruses producing encephalitis, or inflammation of the brain, may damage the basal ganglia and cause Parkinson's disease. In the 1920s there was a worldwide epidemic of a disease called encephalitis lethargica ("sleepy sickness") or von Economo disease. Some victims died, and many survivors were left in a rigid, immobile state, very much like that associated with severe Parkinson's disease. Some people who recovered from the encephalitis developed Parkinson's disease many years later. The name *postencephalitic Parkinson's disease* was given to this condition because it differs somewhat from typical Parkinson's disease. We still see rare cases of encephalitis that produce a late Parkinson's syndrome.

# Clinical Features of Parkinson's Disease

The clinical diagnosis of Parkinson's disease is based on abnormalities of movement. A neurologist looks for tremor causing trembling of the hands, stiffness when walking or rotating the wrist, and loss of facial expression. There are few if any tests that help neurologists to confirm the diagnosis, though they usually order an MRI scan of the brain to make sure that no other condition is causing the symptoms. A dopamine PET scan is too expensive, and the changes too late, for this test to be used for the diagnosis of Parkinson's disease.

The typical patient with Parkinson's disease is a man in his sixties who develops a tremor in one hand and starts limping. Men are affected slightly more frequently than women. The tremor occurs particularly when the person is at rest—for instance, just sitting in a chair—and affects the finger and thumb. It is called a pill-rolling tremor because, in the days before mechanization, medication pills were rolled by hand with a similar movement of the finger and thumb.

Over the first few years of the disease, the patient's walking typically becomes slower and more shuffling. The patient has very slow movements, he has very little facial expression, and he blinks his eyes less frequently than normal. This diminished facial expressiveness is called masked facies. When he walks he is somewhat stooped, his steps are

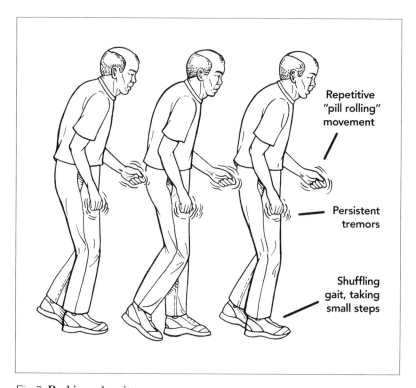

Repetitive "pill rolling" movement

Persistent tremors

Shuffling gait, taking small steps

*Fig. 7:* **Parkinson's gait**

Parkinson's disease produces a stooped posture, shuffling gait and 'pill-rolling' tremor.

small, and his arms do not swing normally. The muscle tone in his limbs is increased when the doctor tries to move them, and this increased muscle tone has a ratchet-like quality called cogwheel rigidity. His writing is tremulous, and for an unknown reason it becomes very small (this is called micrographia).

One paradoxical feature of Parkinson's disease is that, although patients are slow when making a voluntary movement, they can move very quickly if an emergency arises. Neurologists tell medical students a story to drive this point home. The story goes that there was a chronic care facility where many Parkinson's patients lived. Most could not move without a great deal of assistance from the nursing aids. One day the nurses discovered a fire and rang the fire alarm. As soon as the Parkinson's disease patients heard this, they all jumped out of their chairs and ran outside. When they reached safety, the Parkinson's disease kicked in again and they just stood there, immobile. You can demonstrate this phenomenon by tossing a ball to a patient with Parkinson's disease; he will react quickly and catch it. However, when he is asked to throw the ball back, his voluntary movements are so slow that he cannot throw it.

As Parkinson's disease progresses, walking becomes slower and the patient finds it difficult to get his feet moving. Because the patient's feet seem to be stuck to the floor by magnets, this phenomenon is called a magnetic gait. The patient often has to do a little dance to get his feet moving before being able to initiate the first step. He may stop at a threshold such as a doorway and be unable to walk through it. In addition, the patient's voice is often softer (this is called hypophonia), and his speech is monotonous, rapid, and indistinct.

Parkinson's disease does not look the same in every patient. The clinical signs vary greatly. Some patients have no tremor and are just rigid and slow. Others have only tremor, with little or no slowness. In some people the disease affects only one side of the body (called hemi Parkinsonism).

The rate of progression of the disease also varies greatly. Some patients reach an advanced stage of disability within five years, while others remain only mildly affected ten years after the first signs of the disease appeared. Some patients have signs of other neurological conditions in addition to pure Parkinson's disease, particularly in the later stages. Slowness of mind and dementia can occur, as can problems of eye movement and control of blood pressure and bladder. I will describe these conditions later in this chapter, in the section on other movement disorders.

# Treatment and Prognosis of Parkinson's Disease

In the old days, before we had any treatment for Parkinson's disease, the symptoms might progress to total immobility and eventual death from any one of the problems of the aged, such as pneumonia, heart attack, or cancer. The treatment of Parkinson's disease has advanced dramatically in the last forty years as a result of Hornykiewicz's discovery that the brains of patients with Parkinson's disease are deficient in dopamine. This led George Cotzias, a Greek-born physician-neuroscientist working at Brookhaven National Laboratory in New York, to treat patients with L-dopa. This chemical is the precursor of dopamine, meaning that the substantia nigra neurons use L-dopa to make dopamine.

Cotzias found that some patients responded dramatically to the new treatment, but other neurologists were not convinced. Finally scientists realized that patients needed a much higher dose of L-dopa than was used initially. We now know that L-dopa produces a dramatic benefit in patients with Parkinson's disease by increasing the amount of dopamine released at the nerve terminals of the remaining substantia nigra neurons.

Many people have read Oliver Sacks's wonderful book *Awakenings* (1973) or have seen the movie of the same name. Sacks used the then-experimental drug L-dopa to treat patients with postencephalitic Parkinson's disease and observed an almost miraculous response.

In the late 1960s, I was involved in some of the earliest United Kingdom trials of L-dopa to treat Parkinson's disease. I well remember one woman who came to the clinic on a stretcher because Parkinson's disease made her unable to walk. She was only forty but looked twenty years older. She was markedly obese and immobile, and I could hardly hear her because her voice was so soft. She did have a little tremor, but her slowness of movement and frozen face were the most striking signs of Parkinson's disease. She joined our trial of L-dopa. We were kept from knowing which patients received the drug and which received a placebo, but when she walked into the clinic three months later it was clear that she was getting the active drug. She was wearing makeup, had lost ten pounds, and looked twenty years younger. She was cooking for her husband, looking after the house, and getting back to being the vigorous homemaker that she had been five years earlier.

Over time we have learned that if L-dopa alone is taken by mouth, most of it is metabolized in the liver and never reaches the brain. This metabolism can be blocked by a chemical called carbidopa, which has too large a molecule to cross the blood vessel wall into the brain (the blood-brain barrier). Carbidopa blocks the destruction of L-dopa in the liver, thus allowing larger amounts of the medication to enter the brain to be made into dopamine.

Originally, we hoped that L-dopa would totally cure Parkinson's disease. Unfortunately, that proved not to be the case. We now know that progressive degeneration of the substantia nigra neurons continues despite L-dopa treatment. While L-dopa increases the amount of dopamine in the basal ganglia, thereby masking the loss of the substantia nigra neurons for a period of time, it does not cure the underlying disease. L-Dopa begins to lose its effect when the disease is advanced. Patients at this stage suffer from the "on-off phenomenon," where they suddenly go from being mobile to being "frozen" or vice versa. This can be very dangerous if the patient is crossing the road or driving.

When Parkinson's disease has advanced to the stage when only a few substantia nigra neurons remain, L-dopa therapy causes twisting, contorting movements called dyskinesias. You would expect patients who are writhing in a chair due to dyskinesias to be very uncomfortable and want the drug stopped. However, they always insist that they do not want their dose of anti-Parkinson's drugs to be reduced, because they prefer these abnormal movements to being completely immobile.

Since the introduction of L-dopa forty years ago, scientists have developed many new drugs that work on the dopamine receptor directly, thus bypassing the need for substantia nigra neurons to make dopamine. These direct-acting agonists, as they are called, offer additional weapons in the fight against the symptoms of Parkinson's disease.

## Prognosis of Parkinson's disease

As I have pointed out, Parkinson's disease is variable in its rate of development. Some patients have mild signs of Parkinson's disease but do not progress to severe disability. In others, particularly when the disease develops in a person's younger years, it tends to progress more rapidly. We do not understand the reason for this variability, which makes it impossible for a neurologist to forecast accurately what is going to happen to a patient at the time of diagnosis. It is therefore important for neurologists to tell a newly diagnosed patient that progressive disability and early death are by no means the inevitable consequences of Parkinson's disease.

## Neurosurgical treatment of Parkinson's disease

Neurosurgeons became interested in Parkinson's disease when it was observed that a stroke in a Parkinson's patient abolished the tremor. They began making small areas of damage (lesions) in the area of the brain that had been affected by this stroke. By trial and error, the neurosurgeons found that lesions in the thalamus and basal ganglia were most effective for stopping the tremor. However, these neurosurgical procedures did not improve most of the other features of Parkinson's disease, such as slowness and rigidity.

More recently, scientists have developed a new treatment for Parkinson's disease. It is called deep brain stimulation (DBS). Fine wire electrodes are implanted into the deep parts of the brain. The electrodes can be stimulated with a pacemaker embedded under the skin of the chest. The stimulator may be programmed with an external magnet to provide the optimum response.

DBS can bring about dramatic improvement in patients with parkinsonian and essential tremor (see below), as well as in those with dopamine-induced dyskinesias. It is very rewarding to see writhing dyskinesias and wild tremors cease when the stimulator is turned on. More than 40,000 patients worldwide have had DBS implants. Eventually the procedure may be found to help patients with other neurological diseases, such as pain syndromes and cerebellar ataxia, if the electrodes are placed in appropriate areas of the brain.

## Stem cells and Parkinson's disease

Great excitement broke out in the 1980s, when doctors reported apparently successful treatment of Parkinson's disease by putting portions of the patient's own adrenal glands into the basal ganglia. These studies used adrenal cells that secrete dopamine, but the technique eventually was shown not to work. Later, however, implants of embryonic dopamine-producing neurons from aborted human fetuses did survive and produce some improvement, but these neurons did not integrate correctly into the circuitry of the basal ganglia, and most patients developed uncontrollable dyskinesias.

These results highlight the obstacles that stem cell research must overcome to be able to treat brain diseases effectively. Successful treatment will require stem cells to be accurately placed. The cells must develop into neurons that become hardwired into the patient's neuronal network. When in place and connected, the stem cells have to stop proliferating; otherwise they will produce a tumor. So far, scientists have been unable to overcome all of these hurdles to cure degenerative neurological diseases like Parkinson's disease through use of stem cells.

# Other Types of Movement Disorders

The term *movement disorder* could be applied to any neurological condition affecting movement, such as stroke, spinal cord injury, or peripheral nerve or muscle disease. However, neurologists use the term for a specialized group of conditions *without* any of these causes. Parkinson's disease, essential tremor, and several other well-recognized conditions are classified as movement disorders. They can be diagnosed by an experienced neurologist, and treatment is available for some. Conditions that look a little like Parkinson's disease, but have additional features, are called Parkinson-plus syndromes.

## Essential tremor

People who develop a little tremor of the hands often become terrified of developing Parkinson's disease. Usually, however, the tremor is caused by a much more benign condition variously called benign essential tremor, benign familial tremor (since it often runs in families), or benign senile tremor (since it tends to come on in later life). Benign essential tremor is so named because it is not accompanied by any of the degenerative features in conditions like Parkinson's disease. However, the tremor itself does tend to worsen as the decades go by.

Essential tremor has a frequency of six to twelve cycles per second. This is the same frequency as that of the physiological tremor associated with anxiety, caffeine, and an overactive thyroid gland. The frequency of a Parkinson's-related tremor is about four to six cycles per second. Essential tremor is most obvious when patients are using their hands or holding them outstretched. Some patients experience shaking of the head, called titubation, and sometimes they have a tremulous voice. It is quite common for some members of one family to have marked tremor and others to have very little.

The cause of essential tremor is still not understood. No brain pathology has been recognized. Essential tremor may be a disorder of neurotransmitters or their receptors in the basal ganglia. Two drugs are of some help in reducing the degree of tremor: primidone (Mysoline®) and propranolol (Inderal®). Because both drugs have a sedative effect, most patients do not use them.

Interestingly, a small dose of alcohol suppresses essential tremor for a short time. In Britain we used to say to a patient with essential tremor, "If the Duchess is coming to tea, take a glass of sherry beforehand to prevent the tea cup rattling on the saucer." There is an interesting interplay between alcohol and tremor. Since chronic alcoholics often develop a tremor, a patient with benign essential tremor is sometimes thought to be an alcoholic. Though essential tremor is not caused by alcoholism, the incidence of chronic alcoholism in patients with essential tremor is higher than that of the general population, probably because some use alcohol regularly to suppress the tremor.

The dramatic effect of deep brain stimulation on benign essential tremor is gratifying. DBS is now the established treatment for the small number of people with profoundly debilitating tremor.

## Parkinson-plus syndromes

Neurologists like to restrict the term *Parkinson's disease* to the pure condition and use the term *parkinsonism* or *Parkinson-plus syndrome* for situations where features seen in pure Parkinson's disease are also associated with evidence of degeneration of other parts of the nervous system. I will mention only a few of these, because they are relatively rare.

A patient with progressive supranuclear palsy (PSP) usually complains of problems with his eyes and frequent falls. Neurologists will find that he has staring eyes, with the lids often drawn widely open, and that the eyes do not move when the patient is asked to look in a particular direction. The patient may have difficulty following the doctor's finger in any direction. However, if the doctor holds his finger straight in front of the patient and then moves the patient's head upward, downward, or sideways, then the patient's eyes move involuntarily to stay fixed on the finger. Neurologists call this a supranuclear problem of eye movement. This means the problem lies not in the eye muscles or the cranial nerves that move the eyes, but rather in the connections from the brain to the brain stem neurons that control the cranial nerves.

Multiple system atrophy (Shy-Drager syndrome) is a disease causing degeneration of several parts of the autonomic nervous system. The main symptoms are loss of control of blood pressure when standing (orthostatic hypotension), loss of control of the bladder, and some signs of parkinsonism.

Diffuse Lewy body disease, which I discussed in Chapter 2, is usually characterized by features of parkinsonism and a progressive dementia with early hallucinations.

Corticobasal degeneration characteristically causes difficulty making well-learned movements (apraxia), the alien hand syndrome that I described in Chapter 1, and parkinsonism.

## Huntington's disease

This familial disease was named after George Huntington, the physician son of a doctor in East Hampton on Long Island, New York, who studied his father's patients and wrote several papers about them in medical journals in the 1870s. Huntington's disease is dominantly inherited: one of the parents has the disease, and half of the couple's children are likely to inherit it.

Signs of Huntington's disease, which appear in the middle years of life, include twitches and jerks called chorea. Initially these movements look like simple fidgeting, but eventually the abnormal movements become wilder and the diagnosis is clear. A choreic movement looks like a fragment of an intentional movement, though it is involuntary. The late folk singer Woody Guthrie is perhaps the most famous Huntington's chorea patient. Some patients with Huntington's disease make movements that are more writhing; this is called athetosis.

Other unfortunate manifestations of Huntington's disease include changes in behavior, such as impulsiveness and aggression; changes in mood, particularly depression; and the gradual development of dementia. Patients progress from the first symptoms to total disability in five to ten years. Children who have seen a parent go through the progressive degeneration live in fear that they will get the disease. Several of my patients committed suicide from fear of the disease or recognition that they were developing early signs of the condition.

Huntington's disease is caused by degeneration of neurons in the caudate nucleus—a part of the basal ganglia deep in the brain—and in the cerebral cortex. After many years of diligent work, researchers identified the gene responsible for this condition, and the protein it produces was named huntingtin. The mutation causes an excess amount of DNA in one part of the gene. This excess DNA is in the form of too many triplet repeats of bases that make up the genetic code, and these repeats translate into too many molecules of the amino acid glutamine in one region of the huntingtin protein. The increased number of glutamine molecules makes the protein become "sticky," form into clumps in the neurons of the caudate nucleus, and in doing so poison the neurons. Exactly how this mutant protein kills the neurons is still uncertain, and until we know this we will not be able to effectively treat or arrest the disease.

Currently, we have no way to prevent the development or fatal progression of Huntington's disease. Treatment can only relieve symptoms through drugs that decrease the chorea, such as haloperidol (Haldol®) or tetrabenazine (Xenazine®). Depression is a significant side effect of these drugs, particularly tetrabenazine.

We can now offer genetic counseling and a DNA blood test to siblings and children of patients with Huntington's disease. This can help them avoid passing the gene to their children. Unfortunately, a positive test reveals that the subject also has inherited the gene and is therefore likely to develop the disease. When faced with this dilemma, about half the at-risk family members decide that they would not be able to live with this information and decide not to have the test. The other half decides that they have the strength to live with the knowledge that they have the gene mutation. They want to know so that they can decide how to adjust their lives. Follow-up studies of the 50 percent who decided to have the test have shown that, even if the test was positive, most were glad they had the test done.

People who have the Huntington's mutation can have children who are free of the risk of inheriting the gene. They can do this through adoption, artificial insemination by donor (AID), or in vitro fertilization. In the latter procedure, the egg and sperm of the couple, one of whom has the mutant gene, are united outside the body. The embryos are allowed to develop to the sixteen-cell stage, and then one cell is taken for DNA analysis (this is called preimplantation embryonic cell sampling). If the embryo has the mutated gene, it is discarded. Only embryos with the nonmutated huntingtin gene are implanted into the mother's uterus. This procedure is expensive, but it should ensure that children of a parent with Huntington's disease will not be at risk.

## Wilson's disease

We completely understand the biochemical cause of Wilson's disease, which means we can treat this movement disorder. In Wilson's disease, an inherited abnormal gene for copper metabolism causes excessive copper deposition in the brain. Copper is a normal trace element in our diets and is essential for many biochemical processes in our cells. It is normally absorbed through the intestine, and excess is excreted in the bile. Most Wilson's cases result from inability to excrete excess copper in the bile.

The excess copper in the blood of patients with Wilson's disease is first deposited in the liver causing cirrhosis. This is the condition where chronic injury to liver cells causes fibrosis. The excess copper in the blood also becomes deposited in the brain. There it damages the basal ganglia and causes a tremor that makes a patient's outstretched hands flap, as well as an unsteady walk. The excess copper also damages the cerebral cortex, which results in psychiatric manifestations such as childlike behavior and dementia. Copper may also be deposited around the edge of the cornea of the eye, where it produces an appearance called a Kayser-Fleischer ring. Neurologists can detect this ring with a magnifying glass.

The diagnosis of Wilson's disease is based on finding excess copper in the blood and urine, as well as deficiency of the copper-carrying protein ceruloplasmin in the blood. Symptoms usually appear when a person is a teenager or young adult.

Researchers have developed treatments to remove excess copper from the body. The first effective treatment was a diet containing low amounts of copper, plus a foul-tasting, sulfide-containing medication that precipitated the copper in the gut, thereby lowering the amount of copper available for absorption. Later, penicillamine became the standard treatment; it binds the copper and lets the body excrete it. However, penicillamine may cause significant side effects, particularly the triggering of autoimmune diseases. More recently scientists have discovered better treatments, including molybdate and zinc, which compete with copper for absorption from the gut. Zinc therapy is now the standard and best tolerated treatment.

The key to curing Wilson's disease is early diagnosis before significant brain damage has occurred. Once the copper has damaged the brain, though treatment may arrest the disease, only moderate recovery can be expected. The disease is inherited in an autosomal recessive fashion, which means that about a quarter of the siblings may be affected, though the parents are unaffected. If one individual in a family develops Wilson's disease, it is very important to test siblings for early signs of the condition or for low ceruloplasmin blood levels. If others are found to have inherited the disease, they can be treated and saved from neurological damage.

## The dystonias

*Dystonia* literally means "abnormal tone." Patients with dystonia have an incorrect balance of nerve impulses running from the brain to the muscles. This causes abnormal positioning of the limbs or body. The most common form is focal dystonia, which affects a single portion of the body. For instance, spasmodic torticollis is a condition in which the head is usually turned to one side, though it may be twisted in any direction. In other focal dystonias, an arm or a leg may be held in an abnormal posture while the patient walks (this is called limb dystonia), or the eyes may close involuntarily, a condition called blepharospasm.

The term *torsion dystonia* implies that the body is twisted into abnormal postures. Early on in the disease, a patient experiences episodic turning movements. For instance, the arm may be twisted behind the back repeatedly, or the head may be drawn to one side. In the end, the abnormal postures often become fixed. Overactivity of muscles and stretching of ligaments make torsion dystonia a painful condition. We do not know the cause of the disturbed coordination of nerve impulses to muscles.

The first focal dystonia to be attacked surgically was spasmodic torticollis, in which the head and neck are drawn into various positions involuntarily. Several destructive procedures were undertaken to remove or block the nerve connection to the neck muscles or to weaken the muscles that cause the head to turn. The current treatment is to weaken these muscles with botulinum toxin injections that partially paralyze the junction between the nerve endings and the muscles, thus reducing the movements. The paralyzed nerve endings recover in three months. Although repeated injections are needed, botulinum treatment is a major advance for the treatment of dystonias.

Within the group of focal dystonias are conditions labeled as occupational dystonias, though the better term is *task-specific apraxias*. The most common is writer's cramp. Typically, when the patient tries to write, his hand stiffens and shakes. It then grips the pen forcefully and digs it into the paper. Many of us have a very mild form of this condition without realizing it. Our signature is an overlearned motor action that sometimes does not flow correctly. Trying to execute the signature correctly, we tend to tighten our muscles, which makes the signature look different from our typical legal signature. The way to get around this and bring the signature back to normal is to slow down and relax.

Patients with task-specific apraxias often cannot prevent them voluntarily in this way.

Before focal dystonia was well recognized, I had several patients who would now be treated successfully with botulinum injections. Unfortunately, at that time several of them were diagnosed as suffering from hysteria. One was a very successful professional violinist. Suddenly, he began to find that his right (bow) hand went into an overflexed posture whenever he had a difficult piece to play. At first he thought he had had a stroke, but a neurologist found no evidence of this. The neurologist suggested that the violinist had a hysterical condition (or conversion reaction) and referred him to a psychiatrist. A person with a conversion reaction is supposed to obtain some gain from the reaction, in this case the overflexion of the right hand. I could not discern that he had anything to gain and, indeed, he had everything to lose from this problem. Moreover, his hand functioned perfectly normally in every other complex action except for playing the violin. He told me that his only stress was the effect his hand problem was having on his career as a violinist.

Another patient was an avid golfer whose putting had deteriorated suddenly. As he began the smooth swing of the putter, his arm would suddenly jerk, causing him to mis-hit the ball. He got more and more frustrated by this, and one day, in a fit of anger, he struck the golf ball backhanded toward the hole 10 yards away. The ball went in! Since that day, he has putted backhanded, and not suffered any arm jerks. This effective switch of technique clearly demonstrated that task-specific apraxias are movement disorders and not caused by hysteria.

It seems likely that task-specific apraxias arise when one or more parts of the motor memory mechanisms in the nervous system—perhaps the basal ganglia or cerebellum—become dyscoordinated. How and why this happens remains a mystery. The specific motion is always an over-learned one, commonly related to the individual's occupation or avocation, and when the apraxia appears, it cannot be corrected easily. In the past, therapists taught patients to use their hands in a different way to overcome the problem, like my golfer who putted backhanded. More recently, doctors have found some success injecting botulinum toxin into the affected muscles. These injections slightly weaken the muscles and presumably alter the feedback into the motor memory circuits, thus allowing them to reset the overlearned movement.

While neurologists may see focal dystonias from time to time, it is rarer for a patient to appear with one of the familial generalized dystonias. These tragic dystonias are usually dominantly inherited, passing from an affected parent to half of his or her children. The degree of abnormal tone and distortion of the body can be quite profound in these patients. I was the neurologist of several members of a family with generalized dystonia in upstate New York. One of them was confined to a wheelchair in a totally contorted pretzel-like state and had a great deal of resultant pain. Very high doses of diazepam (Valium®) helped relieve the spasms and reduce the pain, so I provided him with the necessary prescriptions. This led to my receiving a visit from a drug enforcement agent who thought that I was giving the patient too many prescriptions and that he was selling the drug on the street. I was eventually able to convince him that patients with this rare disease really need 100 milligrams of diazepam a day to keep their spasms under control.

## Kinesigenic dyskinesia

The rare condition of kinesigenic dyskinesia is perhaps the most bizarre movement disorder I have ever seen. Patients who have it are usually thought to be hysterical. John was in his late teens. His family doctor in rural Vermont sent him to me with a note saying that John seemed to be having seizure attacks, but they did not produce loss of consciousness. John was very shy, and it was difficult to get a good history. He found the attacks very embarrassing. I asked him what they were like, and all he would say was, "I just seem to spasm up."

When I asked John if he could bring on an attack, he got up from the chair, walked a couple of steps, and then dropped to the floor with one knee pulled up to his chest and one arm wrapped around the back of his head. His face was contorted, but he was quite awake. After ten seconds or so the attack passed. He got up from the floor and sat on the chair again.

This seemed to break the ice, and John began telling me his story. The attacks had started when he was about twelve. They would often happen when he was under stress, particularly when he was on a date with a girl. He said that most of the attacks were not as violent as the one that I had witnessed. During the little attacks he could often make it seem like he had reached down to tie his shoe. The attacks eventually led to him become socially isolated, and he was convinced he was possessed by the devil.

Kinesigenic dyskinesia is thought to originate in the basal ganglia, though some neurologists have considered it a form of seizures and given it the name *kinesigenic epilepsy*. The recommended treatment is carbamazepine (Tegretol®). When I gave this to John, the attacks completely disappeared. I saw him several times after that, and he had become an outgoing young man with an active social life.

## The cerebellar ataxias

Disorders of the cerebellum lead to abnormal control of movements, termed ataxia. The cerebellum was originally thought to be simply a fine controller of limb movements, but we now know that it plays a much more complicated role. It stores the templates for movements, called motor engrams, so that a relatively simple command from the higher levels of the brain—such as "Walk!"—is translated into the complex series of integrated muscle contractions required for walking.

Many diseases can damage the cerebellum. Structural problems, such as tumors, abscesses, and hemorrhages, may interfere with the performance of the cerebellum. Inherited conditions called familial cerebellar degenerations can cause an unsteady gait and associated problems with walking over rough ground, turning, and dancing. The disease slowly spreads to the upper limbs, and the patient's hands become unsteady when she writes, picks things up, or puts on makeup.

Eventually her speech becomes slurred. Many patients with cerebellar degeneration eventually become confined to a wheelchair.

The cerebellum may also be damaged by antibodies produced either spontaneously (autoimmune cerebellar degeneration) or in response to the presence of a cancer (paraneoplastic cerebellar degeneration). In Chapter 9, I will describe a patient with the latter.

Toxins can also cause cerebellar dysfunction. In the 1950s, an outbreak of cerebellar ataxia occurred around Minamata Bay in Japan. It was caused by the release of organic mercury compounds from a chemical factory into the waters of the bay. The methyl mercury got into the fish, which local residents then ate. The mercury damaged the cerebellums and peripheral nerves of these patients, eventually leading to permanent severe disability.

Alcohol is another toxin that may damage the cerebellum. Anyone who has been drunk recognizes the slurred speech and unsteadiness that come from intoxication. These signs are caused by inhibition of the cerebellum. Chronic exposure to frequent high doses of alcohol may destroy the cerebellar neurons, particularly the giant Purkinje cells that play a major role in cerebellar function. I had an interesting insight into this condition when I saw a woman with a progressive cerebellar degeneration that had been developing over three or four years. She was unsteady when walking and had slight slurring of speech. I thought that she probably had an idiopathic condition—that is, without a known cause.

As part of my routine inquiry about potential drug toxicity, I asked her if she was taking any regular medication, if she was exposed to unusual chemicals, and if she drank alcohol. To the last question her husband replied, "Yes, we both drink moderately."

"How much do you drink?" I asked.

"Well, we have two or three cocktails a night and maybe a bottle of wine as well. But that can't be the cause, since I drink about the same amount as she does and I don't have problems walking."

This was not necessarily true; though he and his wife were about the same size, different people metabolize drugs differently. I therefore asked her to cut down gradually the amount of alcohol she drank over the next three weeks and then to stop drinking completely for three months. I reduced her intake of alcohol slowly because if people dependent on alcohol suddenly stop drinking, they may have severe withdrawal reactions, including seizures (often called DTs, for delirium tremens).

When my patient came back three months later, she told me that she had stopped drinking completely, and I was surprised to find that her cerebellar ataxia was dramatically better. Her only major residual problem was difficulty walking in a straight line, which is part of the sobriety test used by police. Her husband was so gratified by her improvement that he had greatly reduced his own alcohol intake. These people were not alcoholics in the sense that they were dependent on or addicted to alcohol. They were more like social drinkers. Nevertheless, the wife clearly had difficulty metabolizing alcohol, and it had damaged her cerebellum.

A number of other nervous system diseases cause a cerebellar ataxia in addition to other neurological abnormalities. The most common is Friedreich's ataxia, one of the inherited spinocerebellar ataxias. Patients with this condition suffer from degeneration of the peripheral nerves, the spinal cord, and the cerebellum. Friedreich's ataxia is an autosomal, recessively inherited disease, meaning that although parents are unaffected, one-quarter of the brothers and sisters may also have the same disease. Signs of Friedreich's ataxia begin between the age of nine and sixteen and include unsteady walking and slurring of speech. Patients are often confined to a wheelchair by the end of their teens. The heart also suffers progressive damage in many patients.

We now know that the gene that is mutated in Friedreich's ataxia normally produces a protein called frataxin, which plays a major role in iron metabolism. The mutation leads to iron overload in the tissues, and this interferes with the metabolism of the mitochondria. Though we still do not completely understand how iron overload causes degeneration of the cerebellar Purkinje cells and other parts of the nervous system, medications to reduce the iron load of the body are now being studied as treatments of Friedreich's ataxia. This is an example of how understanding the cause of a disease—even if that understanding is incomplete—can lead to treatment and a possible cure.

It is crucial that a neurologist look for any treatable cause before labeling a condition idiopathic, and it is especially important with regards to cerebellar disease. For example, chronic low thyroid activity can cause cerebellar ataxia, and this diagnosis may not be obvious to the neurologist. A simple blood test can lead to thyroid treatment that cures the disease. Vitamin E is important for the metabolism of cerebellar neurons. Several disorders of vitamin E metabolism show up as spinocerebellar ataxia, which can be arrested with high-dose vitamin E therapy. One of these disorders, abetalipoproteinemia, causes malabsorption of fat and fat-soluble vitamins, including vitamin E, from the gut. A neurologist can recognize the disorder by detecting two things: the presence of spiked red blood cells called acanthocytes in a blood smear and a low vitamin E level.

Deficiency of coenzyme Q10, which is a widely known health food supplement, is also a rare cause of cerebellar degeneration. I have a patient in his early thirties who had an advanced spinocerebellar ataxia. He was bedridden, could not use his hands because they were so unsteady, and was virtually unable to communicate because of his slurred speech. I thought that he might have a mitochondrial disease, so I sent him to colleagues in New York, who did a muscle biopsy. They found that he had a low muscle coenzyme Q10 level, and we started treating him with extremely high doses of coenzyme Q10. He is now able to stand with assistance, use a computer, and communicate well enough to work in a sheltered workshop.

## Chapter 7

# Head Injury

C hildren fall and hit their heads all the time. Parents often worry that their child has suffered a permanent brain injury and will never be the same again. That fear never goes away. Mothers of adult patients with a neurological problem will often say to me, "You know, he fell on his head when he was a baby. Do you think that caused his problem?" Patients who suffer a significant head injury generally ask, "Have I wrecked my brain?" Although the answer to these questions is usually no, in this chapter I will try provide you with an understanding of the mechanism of brain injury, how it is treated, and its prognosis.

LeRoy was a twenty-three-year-old who loved fast cars and prided himself on being a good driver. He also liked to drink with his buddies. After a night out with the boys, he was driving home when another sports car pulled alongside him and then accelerated away. Not to be outpaced, LeRoy stepped on the gas. A traffic light turned yellow as the other car went through an intersection, but LeRoy was not going to be beaten by a mere traffic light. He barreled through the red light and hit a car that had started across the intersection from the right. The driver of that car was killed, and LeRoy went through the windshield of his car; he had not buckled his seat belt.

The ambulance arrived seven minutes later. People were clustered around LeRoy, who was lying in the middle of the intersection. He was unconscious and bleeding from gashes to his face, but he was still breathing. The EMTs put an airway into his mouth. This is a tube that goes down behind the tongue to make sure that the patient is able to breathe. They put LeRoy on a stretcher and took off for the hospital, with lights flashing and horns blaring. My hospital is a Level 1 trauma center, and within two minutes of LeRoy's entering the ER, a trauma surgeon, a nurse, and a medical student all were examining him.

The trauma team found that LeRoy's limbs were not broken, and he did not seem to have any major injury to his chest or abdomen. They assessed his level of consciousness and did a quick neurological examination to see how his brain was functioning. Within five minutes, they had drawn blood and urine to check all his bodily systems and to determine if he had alcohol or illicit drugs in his system that might be relevant to his immediate medical care, and they had set up an intravenous line in a vein in his arm. They then took him to the radiology suite for X-rays of his bones, particularly his spine. From there he was rushed to the CT scanner for a brain scan. The medical student went with him to make sure that LeRoy did not stop breathing. The CT scan showed no skull fracture, but some blood could be seen in the frontal and temporal lobes of his brain.

LeRoy was taken to the trauma intensive care unit (ICU), where he remained unconscious for the following five days. During this time, he had an MRI that showed swelling of the brain and additional areas of damage scattered throughout the deep white matter. For several days after LeRoy regained consciousness, he was very drowsy but able to tell the doctors his name and to move all four limbs on command. Gradually he became alert and was able to remember the name of the hospital and the date. However, he remembered nothing from the time he was in the bar with his pals on the night of the crash up to his sixth day in the hospital. LeRoy was suffering from what is called retrograde amnesia, meaning loss of memories before an injury, and posterograde amnesia, meaning loss of memories after the injury.

After a week in the ICU, LeRoy was transferred to the neurosurgical ward, where physical and occupational therapists began to get him out of bed and to get him talking and walking. He was very slow, both mentally and physically. A neuropsychologist tested him and found that he had significant problems in all aspects of brain function. He had difficulty remembering new things and with simple arithmetic and logic problems. His hands were unsteady, and his speech was slow and slurred.

LeRoy clearly was not able to go home or to return to work any time soon. He was transferred first to an acute rehabilitation ward in the hospital and then to a skilled nursing facility. He had daily physical and occupational therapy and psychological treatment to prepare him for independent living.

LeRoy's recovery was slow. Four months after the accident, he was discharged to his parents' home. He went back to his office, where he had worked as a computer programmer, but within an hour it was obvious to him and his boss that he could not cope with the mental processing required. He eventually found a job as a warehouse assistant and continued to live with his parents. He never regained the mental capacity that he had before the accident.

## What Happens in Head Injury

The brain has been known to be vulnerable to injury ever since the first caveman hit an enemy warrior on the head with his club and saw him fall to the ground unconscious. Even so, the brain has some powers of recovery, as illustrated by the improvement that can occur after a major stroke. Though the skull protects the brain from minor head injuries, the brain wobbles around inside the skull like jelly when the head is hit. A violent blow to the head may move the brain so much that it gets damaged when its delicate nerve fibers tear or when it hits the rigid structures inside the skull.

A patient who suffers a mild head injury is said to have a concussion if he experiences some confusion afterward. This can occur whether or not he loses consciousness. People often take a concussion very lightly, but as we'll see it can result in significant damage to the brain.

An open head injury is one in which the skull is penetrated by an object—for instance, an axe or a bullet. A closed head injury is one in which the skull is not penetrated, though the scalp may be lacerated or the skull fractured. LeRoy had a closed head injury.

You might think an open head injury would be worse than a closed one, but that is not always the case. The degree of injury to the brain depends upon the total amount of energy or force dissipated within the brain substance. A closed head injury, like that suffered by LeRoy, can damage the brain so extensively that the patient cannot survive, even with the best efforts of neurosurgeons and intensivists (doctors who work in ICUs). On the other hand, a small-caliber, low-velocity bullet might penetrate the skull but do less damage to the brain than a severe closed head injury. Nevertheless, the more common scenario is that a high-velocity bullet ricochets within the skull cavity, releasing shock waves throughout the brain that will usually kill the patient.

The area of the brain that is damaged is of crucial importance, and no two head injuries are identical. The differences depend upon the region of the brain damaged, the extent of that damage, and secondary influences such as bleeding (causing low blood pressure) or damage to the lungs (causing low blood oxygen levels). The results of other injuries to the body may markedly worsen the severity of brain injury.

If a penetrating head injury damages an exquisitely important area of the brain, it may result in loss of the function located in that area. For instance, if the language areas on the left side of the brain are damaged, the patient may become unable to speak, read, or understand verbal communication. We say that he has aphasia.

The brain stem—the more primitive part of the brain that connects the cerebral hemispheres with the spinal cord—contains all the ascending and descending nerve fibers going to and from the brain. The center for consciousness is also located in the brain stem. Therefore, injury to the brain stem may produce paralysis that may affect only one side (hemiplegia) or both sides (quadriplegia). It may also produce prolonged coma. If the brain stem injury damages the respiratory center, it results in rapid death unless artificial ventilation is started immediately. Brain stem injuries may occur with a closed head injury, particularly a blow to the side of the head that causes severe rotation of the brain.

Every year in the United States, one in a thousand people suffers a significant head injury. Such injuries send 1.5 million Americans to a hospital emergency room; more than 50,000 of them die of the injury, and at least 100,000 suffer permanent disability. The average cost of admitting a head injury patient to the hospital is over $20,000, and the average lifetime cost of caring for a patient with severe traumatic brain injury is at least $250,000. More than five million Americans now live with significant disability from traumatic brain injury. The total cost of head injuries in the United States exceeds $40 billion annually. High-speed motor vehicle crashes are the major cause of severe head injury, and alcohol and drug use are major risk factors for these accidents.

Athletes who play contact sports are at particular risk for head injuries, particularly those involved in football (both American and soccer), ice hockey, and horse racing. Boxing is the one sport in which the object is to injure the brain of your opponent. A knockout in boxing would be called a concussion in any other circumstance. Motorcyclists, bicyclists, and race car drivers are all at major risk of head injury.

# Diagnosing Brain Injury

The most important method of assessing brain injury is a clinical examination by a physician experienced in caring for patients with head injuries. This doctor may be a neurosurgeon, a trauma surgeon, or a neurologist. The examiner will classify the severity of a closed head injury as mild, moderate, or severe.

The Glasgow Coma Scale was invented to assess how a patient is doing at any particular time after a head injury. It measures the best responses in the categories of motor activity (1 is totally unresponsive, and 6 is normal), verbal response (1 is mute, and 5 is normal), and eye opening (1 means the eyes do not open even in response to pain, and 4 is normal). When the scores in each category are added up, the results are interpreted as follows:

- a patient with a *mild* head injury has a Glasgow Coma Score of 13 to 15 immediately after the accident
- a *moderate* head injury patient has a score of 9 to 12
- a patient with a *severe* head injury has a Glasgow Coma Score of 8 or less

As the patient improves with time the Glasgow Coma Score will increase, but the longer the patient remains at a low level, the worse the eventual outcome is likely to be. LeRoy had a score of 5 when the EMTs examined him at the accident site; his score was 8 when he reached the trauma ER.

Doctors use plain X-rays to look for skull and facial fractures, but a CT scan is generally better, as it can also show bleeding and other damage in the brain. LeRoy's CT scan showed bruising in the frontal and temporal lobes, deep to where his head hit first the windshield of the car and then the pavement. The damage directly under the site of the blow is called the coup injury (from the French word for "blow"). Often the brain rebounds after the head has hit (or has been hit by) something and ricochets against the opposite side of the skull, producing what is called a contrecoup injury.

If LeRoy's injury had fractured the temporal bone at the side of the skull, it might have ruptured the artery running through the skull in that area—the middle meningeal artery. This is one of the reasons for doing an emergency CT scan of the brain, since it will show the expanding pool of blood inside the skull. This blood leakage is called an epidural hematoma.

MRI scans are more sensitive than CT scans for showing damage to the brain in patients with closed head injuries, but an MRI takes longer than a CT scan does. Neither the CT nor the MRI can detect what is going on in the brain at a microscopic level after a head injury. In fact, both scans may look normal even when the patient is in a coma because there is diffuse damage to nerve fibers of the brain. The medical name for this is diffuse axonal injury.

LeRoy remained unconscious for five days after the accident, and the trauma ICU doctors arranged for him to have an MRI of the brain to see what was going on inside his skull. The scan showed swelling of the frontal and temporal areas, the places where the original CT scan had shown bleeding. It also showed tiny white spots of increased MRI-signal deep in the brain; these spots marked areas of diffuse axonal injury.

## Clinical Features and Causes of Brain Injury

Closed head injuries range widely in severity. One injury might cause mild confusion followed by complete recovery within an hour, while another might cause a coma lasting for many years. LeRoy's case illustrates a severe injury, and many such patients die. To some extent, the likelihood of death or survival depends on how rapidly emergency treatment is available.

Consider, for instance, a crash at a car racing circuit. A car traveling at 180 mph touches the tail of the car ahead and spins out, hitting the wall of the racetrack head on. EMTs arrive on the scene of the crash within seconds and drag the driver out of the crushed car. He has no pulse, is not breathing, and appears to be dead. The EMTs put an airway down the back of his throat and a mask on his face and pump oxygen into his lungs. After a couple of minutes, he starts to breathe. Drivers on the racing circuit often survive such severe accidents, partly because emergency medical services are immediately available. The situation is not so favorable on the open road, as we will see when discussing the prognosis of head injuries.

Mild head injuries are fairly common in contact sports. Only now are we coming to realize that they can be much more serious than we originally thought.

Picture this: A 140-pound high school quarterback is hit by a 200-pound defensive linebacker just as he is about to throw the football. He is spun around and thrown to the ground, and he hits his head. The players and officials cluster around him. For a few seconds he does not move, but then he begins to stir. He is carried to the sidelines. A couple of minutes later he says, "Where am I?" He tries to get up, and his teammates help him to the bench. Five minutes later he is saying, "I'm OK. I'm OK! Put me back into the game."

There was a time when high school coaches would have allowed this quarterback to go back onto the field as soon as he said he was okay, but now we know that is unwise. Even though he may seem to have recovered, the quarterback's brain does not function normally for some days after a concussion like this. His reflexes are slowed, which makes him more liable to get a second head injury that can be more devastating.

The American Academy of Neurology guidelines for the management of sports-related head injuries divide concussions into three grades. In a Grade I concussion, there is no loss of consciousness, and confusion clears within fifteen minutes. In Grade II, there is no loss of consciousness but it takes more than 15 minutes for the confusion to clear. In Grade III, the player loses consciousness.

The Academy guidelines indicate when an athlete can be allowed to return to a contact sport based on the grade of his concussion. If it was Grade I, then he may return to play when his mental state has cleared. If he has a second Grade I concussion later in the game, he should be pulled from the game and not allowed to play for at least one week after his mental state has returned to normal. Players with a Grade II concussion should be pulled from the game and not allowed to return that day. Players who suffer a Grade II concussion after having a Grade I concussion on the same day should wait at least two weeks after the symptoms have cleared before playing again. Players with a Grade III concussion should not play for at least a week, even if the loss of consciousness lasted only a few seconds; if loss of consciousness lasts more than a minute, they should not play for at least two weeks.

The high school quarterback I mentioned earlier had a Grade III concussion and should be "benched" for at least a week. After returning to play, if he had a second Grade III concussion, then he should avoid contact sports for at least a month after all signs and symptoms of brain dysfunction have cleared. Though the Academy guidelines are designed for sports-related head injuries, they make clear that it is important to avoid blows to the head in everyday life as well.

Multiple head injuries are common in some sports. Two men get into a ring and pummel each other until one falls to the floor and cannot get up to defend himself again. This "sport" is called boxing, though I call it legalized assault and think they are like the Roman gladiators, who were slaves, convicts, and prisoners of war forced to fight to the death for the pleasure of the spectators. Though death is uncommon in modern-day boxing, professional boxers are slaves to the lure of the big purse.

The World Boxing Association safety code allows a professional boxer to be knocked down a maximum of three times in any one round before he is declared the loser. Any boxer who gets knocked out has by definition suffered a Grade III concussion or worse, and he is suspended for sixty days.

Boxers suffer many brain injuries during their careers. The brains of old professional boxers, who might have had three hundred or more fights, suffer from cerebral atrophy and damage to the deep structures. Many old fighters are slowed mentally and physically, and they often have a slow, shuffling walk and slurred speech. This is called the punch-drunk syndrome, and the symptoms make it look like a combination of Alzheimer's and Parkinson's diseases. Professional boxers are at high risk of developing actual Alzheimer's or Parkinson's disease in later life. It has been suggested that boxing caused Muhammad Ali's Parkinson's disease.

Multiple head injuries are not limited to boxing. Professional jockies often suffer head injuries when they are thrown off their horses. Steeplechase jockeys in Britain are liable to become punch drunk from multiple falls over the high fences. You might think that the brains of soccer players would be damaged when they "head" the ball. Though there are cases of soccer professionals becoming punch drunk, it is remarkably rare. This is because the correct technique for heading is to tighten the neck muscles and prevent the head moving when it hits the ball, so that there is none of the swirling of the brain that happens when boxers get punched.

Although a head injury may fracture the skull, the extent of damage to the brain is not related to whether the skull is fractured. For this reason, guidelines for the management of head injury no longer recommend routine X-rays or CT scans. However, a skull fracture may open the cerebrospinal fluid (CSF) to the risk of infection, or it may damage the cranial nerves running from the brain.

One of my patients was directing the driver of a truck to back into a tight parking space. He was standing against a wall as the truck came toward him. He shouted "Stop!" but the truck driver did not hear him, and his head was trapped between the back of the truck and the wall. He told me that he heard his skull crack, though he did not lose consciousness and was unaware of any other problem. The truck driver realized what had happened and drove forward, releasing my patient. He had a terrible headache but otherwise seemed to be all right, until a few days later, when he leaned forward and found clear fluid running from his nose. He initially thought it was mucus from his allergies. However, the fluid continued to pour out whenever he leaned forward, and he came to see me about it. I found that the fluid contained glucose. This proved it was CSF, since nasal mucus does not contain glucose. The truck accident had fractured his skull through the area at the top of the nose. This created a fistula, or pathway, for the CSF to escape into the nasal cavity. The condition is called CSF rhinorrhea, from the Latin meaning "fluid flowing from the nose."

Another patient had suffered a head injury a year earlier. He came to me complaining of a sloshing sound in his head when he moved. X-rays showed that the cavities of his brain were full of air that had been sucked into the skull through a silent skull fracture going through the nasal sinuses. Air in the cavities of the brain (the ventricles) is called pneumocephalus.

Both of these patients were lucky that they did not develop meningitis, which is a common complication of skull fractures that produce communication between the CSF and the nasal cavity. Both injuries required that a neurosurgeon operate to close the fistula.

If a fracture goes through the base of the skull, cranial nerve injury may result. The facial and olfactory nerves are most frequently injured in this way, leading to paralysis of one side of the face or loss of the sense of smell, respectively.

A severe head injury, whether closed or open, may tear blood vessels at the base of the brain or in the brain substance. As a result, blood can leak into the CSF, producing the syndrome of subarachnoid or intracerebral hemorrhage. This is essentially the same as what I describe in Chapter 3.

If a fracture tears the middle meningeal artery as it runs through the thin part of the skull under the temple, an acute epidural hematoma will result. Unless doctors rapidly drain the epidural hematoma, the increased pressure within the skull will cut off blood supply to the brain and the patient will die. While I was doing neurosurgery during my training, I saw a motorcyclist who crashed his bike and hit his head on the road. He was knocked out for a few minutes but then got up from the ground, only to collapse unconscious about ten minutes later. This story of a head injury producing brief loss of consciousness, followed by recovery (sometimes called a lucid interval) and then a loss of consciousness is characteristic of an acute epidural hematoma, and most of these patients do not reach the hospital alive.

Severe head injuries also may cause bleeding into the region between the tough outer covering of the brain, the dura, and the thin inner covering of the brain, the pia-arachnoid membrane. A blood clot in this space is called a subdural hematoma. An acute subdural hematoma results from bleeding in the brain after a severe head injury. On the other hand, a chronic subdural hematoma slowly accumulates over weeks or months after a mild head injury and produces slowly worsening headaches due to rising intracranial pressure. The bleeding comes from ruptured veins that run from the brain to the sagittal sinus—the main draining vein of the brain.

All penetrating head injuries destroy an area of brain, produce hemorrhage, and bring potentially infectious material inside the skull. This may cause meningitis—an infection of the CSF and the meninges (membranes covering the brain)—or the infected material may enter the brain and produce an abscess. A bullet often causes so much damage that severe brain swelling kills the patient. A piece of shrapnel may cause less extensive damage. The patient may eventually recover, and a scar will replace the damaged brain tissue.

A severe closed head injury will produce diffuse axonal injury, with numerous areas of torn nerve fibers, deep in the white matter of the brain and brain stem. Such injury to nerve fibers might not result in complete loss of any single neurological function, but it may cause widespread deterioration of many capacities of the brain. The patient may be left with severe disability because of difficulty in mental processing, memory, and motor coordination.

When any tissue is injured, it swells; the brain is no exception to this rule. The brain has the additional problem of being inside a closed box—the skull—and any swelling of the brain increases the pressure inside the skull dramatically. This tends to prevent the arteries perfusing the brain, thereby restricting the brain's supply of oxygen and glucose. This may be a cause of continuing unconsciousness after a severe head injury.

A swollen brain may also push on other structures inside the skull. Pressure on the third cranial nerve causes a pupil to dilate; doctors take this as an indication that there is critically raised pressure inside the skull. Doctors and nurses often shine flashlights in the eyes of unconscious patients to see if their pupils are equal in size and reactive to light. If a pupil is dilated and unreactive to light, it is an emergency and a neurosurgeon has to open the head and relieve the pressure.

Study of the brain at autopsy has taught us a lot about the damage that results from traumatic brain injury. However, since only the most severely injured patients die, autopsy studies have not shown what happens in patients with milder head injuries. Brain trauma research therefore has to be done on small laboratory animals like rats. Due to the small size of these animals' brains, they may not react exactly like the brains of humans. Studies done on monkeys more than sixty years ago helped illuminate what happens inside the human skull at the time of an acceleration-deceleration injury.

When a fixed head is hit with a padded instrument, most of the energy is concentrated on the brain below the site of the blow and on the opposite side of the brain, and the hit results in coup and contrecoup lesions. However, if the head is free and it rotates as a result of the blow—as when a boxer is punched or when LeRoy was thrown through his windshield—the brain swirls around inside the skull like jelly. It rotates one way and then swishes back the other way. The extent of the movement is surprisingly large, and it is easy to understand how small blood vessels and many axons deep in the brain and brain stem are torn in this process. A rotating blow can be worse than a direct blow from the front because it produces more shearing injury to the long axons.

## Treatment and Prognosis of Brain Injury

Many people with head injuries are much less severely affected than LeRoy; they do not need to be admitted to the hospital, or they are discharged after only a few days. LeRoy's injury was severe, and he was lucky that the accident happened in a big city with a Level 1 trauma center. If he had been injured in the country, it might have taken an hour for an ambulance to reach him, and he might not have survived. The longer the time between the injury and the arrival of medical help, the poorer the outcome—that is, the lesser the degree of recovery of neurological function. The goal of the EMTs is to restore ventilation and blood pressure as rapidly as possible. This is called the ABC of head injury: Airway, Breathing, Circulation. Correcting problems in these areas minimizes secondary damage to the brain from lack of oxygen and low blood pressure.

Once the ABC is taken care of, the emergency crew rushes the injured patient to the nearest hospital emergency department, where he will receive treatment and investigation just like my patient LeRoy. If medical personnel find evidence of a large hemorrhage or severe swelling of the brain, the patient will be taken to the operating room, where neurosurgeons will open his skull to relieve the pressure. If the patient has a lot of brain swelling but not enough to require neurosurgery, he may be given intravenous medications, such as high-dose corticosteroids and a drug called mannitol, to reduce the swelling. He is then taken to the ICU, which provides the modern nursing and medical care necessary to maintain life and to allow the brain to recover as much as possible.

As in the case of a stroke, maintaining normal blood pressure and levels of glucose and oxygen, as well as preventing fever, improve the degree of recovery in a patient with a head injury. Abnormalities of any of these measures make it harder for the injured brain to recover. In some centers, patients or their brains are cooled to try to improve the outcome after severe head injury.

The brain has surprising powers of recovery after injury, though they are not as effective as in organs like the liver, kidney, or muscle. When neurons are injured significantly, they usually die. The brain has almost no capacity to form new neurons. Surviving neurons may sprout, but as I will describe in the next chapter the central nervous system generally prevents axons from regenerating very far.

Experts in the field of neurorehabilitation specialize in helping the brain recover. Therapists of several specialties—physical, occupational, speech, and psychology—work with the patient for several hours a day to try to accelerate the healing process. Their goal is to stimulate the patient's surviving neurons to take over the functions of the neurons that died. Their work is slow and painstaking. The speed of recovery is often frustratingly slow for the patient and his loved ones.

The more severe the head injury and the slower its rate of improvement immediately after the accident, the slower and less effective is the degree of recovery. As the expression goes, "Time is the great healer," and only rehabilitation is known to speed up the process.

A patient with a very severe head injury may never recover conscious-ness and, after a few days, may be shown to have no brain function. We know that such a brain-dead patient has no chance of recovery, and his next of kin will generally agree to withdraw life support once the doctors have explained the prognosis to them.

In some patients, the degree of damage is slightly lower than brain-death, but the patient continues to need life support for months or even years. In this situation, the patient's degree of recovery over time is limited. Some patients in this situation recover consciousness but remain severely mentally and physically handicapped, and they require total care for the rest of their lives. Very few ever return to an independent life.

Some severely injured patients may eventually enter the persistent vegetative state (PVS). These patients recover the primitive functions located in the brain stem, including spontaneous respiration and sleep/wake cycles, but they recover none of the functions of the higher parts of the brain, most importantly the cerebral cortex. They may open their eyes to a loud noise or a touch, and may even follow movements with their eyes, but these are simply reflex responses occurring in the primi-tive parts of the brain. The patients are by definition unconscious since they are unable to have any cognitive interaction with people around them. They have no internally driven behavior, such as moving at will or speaking to say that they are hungry or in pain. Imaging of the brain or autopsy shows severe atrophy of the brain resulting from death of neurons and their axons.

However, when family members see these reflex responses, it is very difficult for them not to believe that their loved one is waking up, though these movements are automatic, just like a knee jerk. Nevertheless, it is important not to diagnose PVS before three months after an anoxic episode, in which the blood to the brain gets cut off for a prolonged period of time, as in a patient whose heart stops. Neither should a neurologist diagnose PVS until at least six months after a traumatic brain injury, like LeRoy's. During these time periods, a few patients do recover some level of consciousness, though very few get anywhere near their mental and neurological state before the brain injury.

I cared for a patient who was one of the lucky ones. A man brought his beautiful wife from South America to see me in Miami because she had anoxic brain injury from a cardiac arrest that had occurred five days earlier during a plastic surgery operation. General anesthesia has a minute risk of causing the heart to stop, and she had drawn the short straw. I just wished that she had not felt the need to have a tummy tuck to return her shape to "normal" after the birth of her last child.

My patient remained unconscious and unresponsive for more than four weeks, and I was fairly certain she was beginning to go into PVS. Her husband kept insisting that she was responding to him, but the nurses and I could find no response to our testing, so I told him that he was seeing reflex reactions that did not indicate recovery of consciousness.

A little later, the nurses started telling me that they thought she was reacting, and again I could not confirm it. I gave them the lecture about it being very difficult to separate a reflex response from an internally driven cognitive action. However, about a week later, even I became convinced that she was making independent motions.

Over the next three months, she gradually returned to being alert, though still with severe neurological damage. She was left with moderately severe spasticity in all four limbs and slowness of speech, but she was able to get around and look after her house and family. She even recovered her bubbly personality, and she and her family were delighted with her recovery.

With good medical care, patients suffering from PVS can live for many years. American heiress, socialite, and philanthropist Sunny von Bülow, whose husband Claus was accused of trying to murder her, slipped into a coma followed by PVS in 1980 and remained in that state for twenty-eight years. Other cases of PVS that caused a great furor in the media and the courts include Karen Ann Quinlan, Nancy Beth Cruzan, and Terri Schiavo in the United States and Alan Bland in the United Kingdom. Their names bring to mind many bitter emotional and legal struggles. Such cases have made adversaries of the medical profession and a good percentage of society on the one hand,

and religious fundamentalists, the right-to-life movement, and those supporting the rights of the disabled on the other. Courts and legislatures have labored long and hard trying to balance opposing views and to allow the right of self-determination to injured individuals and those who hold their durable power of attorney. Because of the difficulties in resolving such opposing views, neurological organizations in the United States set up the Multi-Society Task Force on Persistent Vegetative State to provide guidelines on how to deal with PVS for legislatures and courts.

## Late effects of mild head injuries

The commonest symptoms that occur after a mild head injury are headaches, dizziness, lack of clarity of thought, and depression. This is called post-concussion syndrome. This is a very reproducible collection of legitimate symptoms. However, the frequency of these complaints is much lower in patients who have much more severe brain injuries or sports-related head injuries. It is fairly clear that some individuals who suffer a mild head injury at work or in a traffic accident claim to have post-concussion syndrome because they seek legal compensation. Such symptoms are not necessarily made up, but subconscious or conscious (malingering) exacerbation or perpetuation of symptoms can undoubtedly occur.

Loss of smell is a very frequent effect of mild to moderate head injury. Shaking of the brain may rupture the tiny olfactory nerve filaments running from the receptors that perceive scents, inside the top of the nose, through a perforated part of the skull at the top of the nasal cavity to the olfactory bulb attached to the brain. People who have lost their sense of smell also lose most of their ability to taste food, since appreciation of food is derived from aromas that go up the back of the nose and stimulate receptors for smell. The only taste sensations left for such patients are those of salt, sweetness, bitterness, sourness, and umami (meaty or savory, the taste-enhancement receptors stimulated by MSG) that are perceived by the tongue.

Headaches are a very frequent post-concussion problem and often have many of the features of migraines. Another common post-concussion difficulty is dizziness. This symptom may amount to just a swimming feeling but frequently has a spinning (rotatory vertigo) component, in which the patient has a sudden sense of spinning if he turns his head quickly or turns over in bed. When a doctor tests the effect of the head turning, the patient's eyes will jiggle around in a characteristic picture that we call nystagmus. We believe this comes from problems in the semicircular canals of the inner ear. The head injury shakes loose debris into the fluid in the semicircular canals and damages the hair cells that send their messages to the brain to tell it about head movement. This debris overstimulates the injured hair cells.

Patients frequently complain of being unable to concentrate normally after a significant head injury. They are easily distractible, like a child with an attention deficit syndrome, and short-tempered. They also have poor insight into their condition. This is not due to depression, though depression is common after a significant head injury. Rather, it is due to subtle damage to many pathways in the brain resulting from diffuse axonal injury.

Seizures may occur following head injury. They occur in more than a quarter of patients who suffer a penetrating brain injury that produces a scar on the brain, but they are rare after a closed head injury. Patients may have seizures in the first day or two after injury, but usually there is a prolonged interval between the injury and the first seizure. If the seizures are frequent and unresponsive to antiepileptic medication, it may be possible to remove the scarred area of the brain responsible for the seizures, as I describe in Chapter 4. Removal of the scar may end the seizures, but they may return after a few years.

## Prevention of Head Injuries

Society has a stake in protecting its citizens from head injuries because of the cost of hospitalization, long-term care, and loss of productive lives. We try to reduce injuries and death while driving through improved design of motor vehicles, seat belts and air bags, enforcement of speed limits, and drug and alcohol regulations. Through various laws and guidelines, such as those requiring motorcycle and bicycle riders to wear helmets, we try to protect that most crucial human organ, the brain.

Should we live wrapped in cotton, or should we live a normal life and accept the risk of suffering a head injury when we play sports or drive a car? The answer is fairly clear, but we can take sensible precautions to limit the risk. The brain is our most precious organ, but it is unforgiving. Unlike the body's other organs, the brain has limited power to regenerate. Any recovery that occurs after a severe head injury happens because an undamaged part of the brain has learned a new task and taken on the job of the part of the brain that was damaged.

Chapter **8**

# Spinal Cord Injury

Mario was a twenty-two-year-old naval recruit who planned to go to architecture school after completing his time in the service. He was horsing around with friends when he dove into a swimming pool. Unfortunately, he chose the shallow end of the pool. He hit his head on the bottom, fractured his neck, and suffered a spinal cord injury. The fracture pushed part of his neck vertebra back into the narrow spinal canal that contains the spinal cord, and Mario's spinal cord was crushed. He was immediately unable to move his arms and legs, and he would have drowned if his friends had not been watching. They pulled Mario out of the water and asked him what had happened. All he knew was that he had hurt his neck and could not feel his arms or legs.

His friends called for an ambulance, which arrived ten minutes later. The paramedics quickly realized that Mario had a cervical spinal cord injury. They gently slipped a collar around his neck to prevent movement that could have produced further injury to the spinal cord. Then they slid a board under his back and lifted him onto a stretcher and into the ambulance. They quickly rushed him to the hospital, where the neurosurgery team took over his care.

The neurosurgical resident examined Mario and found that Mario could neither feel anything below the shoulders nor move his arms or legs. His breathing was shallow but adequate. The resident took Mario to the CT scanner and, within ten minutes, knew that he had a fracture of the fifth of the neck's seven vertebrae—this is known as C5. There was a small displaced fragment of bone pushed back into the spinal canal, where it was pushing on the spinal cord.

The neurosurgical team took Mario to the operating room, put him to sleep, and carefully turned him on his front. The operation on the back of his neck was very delicate. Surgeons opened his spine from the back, taking care to avoid doing more damage to the spinal cord, and removed the fragment of bone.

Nowadays, spinal neurosurgeons and orthopedic surgeons work as a team. They put in a rigid titanium device that looks like a G-clamp to hold together the vertebrae above and below the fractured vertebra, thus stabilizing the spinal column and preventing movement around the fractured vertebra. Mario's injury occurred thirty years ago, however. At that time, neurosurgeons inserted a bone graft from the hip region to fuse the spine and kept the patient's neck immobilized in a cervical brace (a very large, rigid collar) for three to six months. After they finally closed everything up, they knew that it was simply a matter of waiting to gauge the recovery of Mario's spinal cord function.

I saw Mario the next day, when he was transferred to my neurology service for rehabilitation. His neurological examination was the same as when the neurosurgical resident first had assessed him. This was reassuring because at least he had suffered no additional damage from the surgery. Mario told me that he had no pain but was terrified about what was going to happen to him. I told him that it was too early to know how much recovery would occur but that it was our job to help him recover as much as we could and get him mobile as soon as possible.

# What Happens in Spinal Cord Injury

It is difficult to imagine how devastating a severe spinal cord injury must be for a young person in the prime of life. One moment he has everything to look forward to, and the next all is lost. He will be confined to a wheelchair for the rest of his life, with loss of sexual function and difficulty controlling his bowels and bladder. At first he does not believe what the doctors are telling him: that he will never be able to walk again. Slowly, as the days pass and he still cannot move or feel his legs, realism dawns and he becomes very depressed. The word *cripple* looms large in his mind.

All of us who care for patients suffering from a spinal cord injury know that the most important gift we have to give is hope. Hope that they will see some recovery over time. Hope that they will be as successful as many who have suffered a spinal cord injury and achieved a happy life. Hope that researchers will find a way to heal the spinal cord injury and cure paralysis.

The spinal cord is well protected by the massive bony structures of the spinal vertebral column, but the cord may still be injured by a bullet or knife. Much more frequently, spinal cord injury results from extreme forces on the spine, such as when a person falls from a height or is involved in a motor vehicle accident. These severe forces cause excessive movement of the head on the neck and trunk; this, in turn, puts so much strain on the cervical spine that often a vertebra fractures. In other cases, one vertebra may slip on the next because the ligaments that secure them are torn. As a result, the spinal cord is squeezed and sometimes completely crushed.

Because it has the greatest mobility and the least strength, the cervical spine in the neck is particularly vulnerable to high-speed motor vehicle accidents and whiplash injuries. Though fractures of the lumbar vertebrae at the bottom of the back are common, the spinal cord extends only to the first lumbar vertebra; below that level a fracture may injure the nerve roots running to the legs and bladder, instead of the spinal cord. Fractures of spinal vertebrae in the area of the shoulder blades, called the thoracic region, can cause damage to the thoracic spinal cord, but they are much less frequent because of the immobility and strength of the vertebral column in that region.

About 12,000 people in the United States suffer a severe spinal cord injury each year, and 200,000 Americans are currently living with some degree of paralysis and disability as a result. Most people with spinal cord injury are between the ages of twenty and forty, and 85 percent of them are men. Motor vehicle accidents cause nearly half the injuries; falls, violence (particularly gunshot wounds), and sports injuries make up most of the remainder. More than half of affected patients have neck injuries. The lifetime cost of medical care of a quadriplegic patient exceeds $2 million. Spinal cord injuries cost the nation $10 billion each year.

## Tests Used in the Investigation of Spinal Cord Injury

The most important "test" for a patient with spinal cord injury is the initial neurological examination. When the EMTs were with Mario beside the swimming pool, they recorded the first examination. The neurosurgical resident who admitted Mario to the hospital conducted the same exam. As in Mario's case, if the patient's neurological signs remain unchanged between these two examinations and during the next couple of days, then the spinal cord injury will likely remain severe. If the patient improves between the first and subsequent examinations, the prognosis for recovery is much better.

When a patient with a suspected spinal cord injury comes into the emergency department, the very first diagnostic test done is usually an X-ray or a CT scan of the injured area. In Mario's case this test centered on the injury to his neck. Plain X-rays would have shown the fracture but would not as readily have shown the bone fragment in his spinal canal. MRI scanners were not available when Mario was admitted with spinal cord injury, but now we use them to show the spinal cord more clearly than on a CT scan. In a case like Mario's, an MRI would have shown that his spinal cord was swollen due to the crush injury at the C5 level next to the fracture.

The important question in someone with a spinal cord injury is whether any of the nerve fibers of the spinal cord have survived: motor nerve fibers running from the brain to move the arms and legs, and sensory nerve fibers running to the brain from the arms and legs. Technicians can do a test called transcranial magnetic stimulation, which fires impulses from the brain down the motor fibers by applying magnetic pulses through the skull to the motor area of the cerebral cortex. If these impulses make the arm and leg on the opposite side of the body move, then at least some part of the spinal cord at the site of injury has survived.

The magnetic stimulator apparatus is available only in a few centers, but there is a similar, somewhat more widely available test called a somatosensory evoked potential study. In this procedure, the sensory nerves in the arms or legs are stimulated with weak electrical currents, and recording electrodes are placed over the sensory cortex of the brain. If the signals of nerve impulses manage to pass through the injured area of the cord to reach the sensory cortex of the brain, then the spinal cord injury is not total.

In the end, the best way to determine whether some nerve fibers have survived the injury—and therefore to forecast the degree of recovery—is to do repeated neurological examinations of the patient. Every day the neurology residents and I examined Mario to see if any movement had returned to his paralyzed limbs, or to find out how far up the body he felt a pinprick (we call this the sensory level.) If these examinations show any improvement, it indicates that nerve fibers that were injured but not destroyed are starting to recover.

## Clinical Features of Spinal Cord Injury

The most frequent location of spinal cord injury is at the fifth and sixth cervical vertebral level, the most mobile part of the cervical spine. A "complete" spinal cord lesion at the C5 level—an injury that has crushed all the nerve fibers passing through that area—will leave the patient able to move his shoulders and flex his arms weakly, but he will lose all motor power and sensation below that level. Thus the patient will be unable to move or feel his hands and legs. A complete spinal cord injury also destroys the nerve fibers that allow the brain to know when the bladder and bowels are full and that control their emptying.

A patient with a complete cervical spinal cord injury has what is termed quadriplegia. Injuries of the thoracic or lumbar cord spare the arms but cause paralysis and numbness of the legs along with incontinence; this is termed paraplegia. Penetrating wounds can cut through just one side of the spinal cord to produce what is called

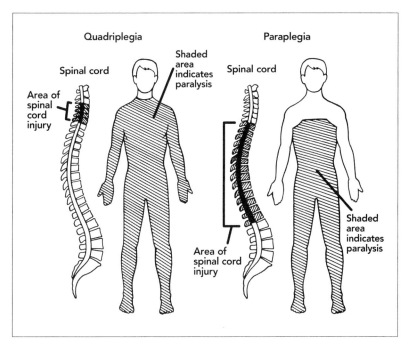

*Fig. 8:* **Paraplegia and quadriplegia**

Loss of movement and sensation occurs from the neck down in quadriplegia from a spinal cord injury in the area of the neck. In paraplegia, the loss takes place downward from a point in the torso, depending on the injury location in the thoracic spinal cord.

Brown-Séquard syndrome. In this condition, movement of the limbs and awareness of the movement of joints in the limbs below and on the same side as the injury are lost, and the sensation of pain and temperature are lost on the side of the body below and opposite to the injury. This strange neurological deficit is the result of the hardwiring pattern in the spinal cord.

Mario awoke from surgery to find that he could still not feel anything below his shoulders, and he could not move his arms or legs. He began to panic because he realized the seriousness of his situation. The nurses tried to calm him, but eventually he needed medication to relax him. Later, he freaked out again when the nurses came to change his urinary catheter. He had not realized that his urine was being drained by a tube in his penis. To have a female nurse deal with his most private part in such a matter-of-fact way was very distressing to Mario, particularly since he could not feel anything.

As the days went by, we began to talk to Mario about what was happening. We told him that his spinal cord had been damaged by the neck fracture, but we did not know how badly. Only time would tell. So far, we had not seen any sign of recovery, but it was still early. In the next three or four weeks, we would have a better idea.

Three weeks after Mario's accident, his sensory level descended slightly to the thumb and he was able to flex his arms at the elbow. This was encouraging to us because it meant that some healing was going on in the fifth and sixth cervical segments of the spinal cord. However, this degree of recovery was of no interest to Mario, who became very depressed. One stupid action had stolen his bright future and had made him a cripple. He saw all his dreams shattered and asked me to let him die. I told him that I certainly could not do that, and that it was far too early to give up hope. I said that the first thing we needed to do was to train his bowels and bladder, because at the moment he was doubly incontinent.

I also pointed out that Mario would get excellent nursing care to prevent bedsores—sometimes called pressure sores or decubitus ulcers—which develop if a paralyzed person lies in one position for too long. If you have normal sensation, you keep shifting your position, thus allowing blood to come back into the skin where it was previously cut off by pressure. If you have no sensation in an area of skin and are paralyzed, unremitting pressure will cut off the blood supply and cause the skin to die.

## Pathology of spinal cord injury

When the spinal cord is injured it may be physically severed all the way across—what we call transected—leaving no connection between the sections of the cord above and below the injury. On the other hand, the cord may be crushed at the level of an injury, but its physical continuity remains intact. In a crush injury, some of the axons that pass through the injured area may survive and eventually regain function. This is called an incomplete lesion. The injured but surviving axons usually do not transmit nerve impulses for days or weeks after the injury, and during this time the patient appears to have a complete spinal cord injury. Slowly the still-intact nerve fibers recover, and some function reappears below the level of the injury. If all the nerve fibers at the crush site have been destroyed, however, the patient has a complete spinal cord lesion. Unfortunately, the only real way to tell if the injury is complete or partial is to wait and see if any recovery of sensation and movement occurs below the level of the injury.

*Spinal cord contusion* is the term for a less severe injury that temporarily distorts the spinal cord but spares most of the axons any permanent injury. Football players who hurt their necks in a game call this injury a burner or a stinger. They feel an acute pain in the neck and an electric-shock sensation down the arms and legs. They may be unable to move, but then they recover in a minute or so. This brief paralysis is a very ominous symptom for any of us who know about spinal cord injury. These players should undergo thorough investigation to make sure that there is no instability of the ligaments and bones of the cervical spine. If I had one of these injuries, I would give up contact sports completely.

The part of a nerve fiber disconnected from its neuron cell body by a spinal cord injury is called the distal axon. When it degenerates it cannot conduct the nerve impulses needed for spinal cord function. In the weeks and months after a spinal cord injury, the natural healing processes of the nervous system gradually remove the damaged tissue at the site of the injury and replace it with scar tissue. Unlike the axons in peripheral nerves, however, axons in the central nervous system do not regenerate. When peripheral nerve axons are cut or crushed, they begin to regrow after a few weeks, and the sprouts eventually make contact with sensory endings or muscles to restore function. That is why surgeons are able to reattach a severed hand, and it will work relatively well when the nerves have regenerated. Although regeneration in the peripheral nervous system is not 100 percent effective, it is certainly better than in the spinal cord.

In some animals, such as the goldfish, axons can regenerate across an injured site in the spinal cord and make the muscles below the injury work as well as before. It might therefore seem that all we need to do to cure spinal cord paralysis is to turn back the clock so that we become goldfish. In fact, humans have not *lost* the capacity to regenerate; instead they have *gained* a new function that prevents regeneration in the central nervous system. It is counterintuitive that more highly developed animals would have developed a new function to make them less versatile, but that is the case.

To understand this, we need to think about the increasingly complex central nervous system as we travel up the animal kingdom until we reach the human. The development of the higher levels of cognition in the cerebral cortex depends upon very complex hardwiring of the branches of neurons—the axons and dendrites—and their contacts, the synapses. Even slight damage to the human brain leads to death of a few of these connections. If the adjacent axons were allowed to sprout to replace the contacts, the hardwiring "diagram" of the central nervous system would become deranged. This would progressively degrade our cognitive capacity and memory processes. The development of mechanisms to *prevent* axonal regeneration may have been the way by which evolution led to the development of human intellect. The central nervous systems of higher organisms, including humans, have a number of proteins—including one evocatively named NOGO—that block the attempts of nerve fibers to regenerate.

# Treatment and Prognosis of Spinal Cord Injury

The ancient Egyptians were well aware of spinal cord injury and its poor prognosis. In the Edwin Smith papyrus—which is thought to have been written about 1800 BCE, based on knowledge dating to 3000 BCE—there is an excellent description of a patient with a fractured neck and spinal cord injury. The papyrus recommends that a physician call this injury an ailment not to be treated (and therefore left to die).

This attitude—that a patient with a spinal cord injury was better off dead and that he would inevitably die—continued through the First World War (1914–1918), in which many soldiers suffered spinal cord injuries and very few survived. Before the era of antibiotics, the paralysis resulting from spinal cord injury led to pneumonia, bladder infections, and pressure sores that festered into blood infections and death. Few patients lived more than two years after sustaining a severe spinal cord injury.

The Second World War (1939–1945) saw a dramatic improvement in the survival of patients with spinal cord injuries. This was due partly to sulfa drugs and penicillin, and partly to the development of the principles of spinal cord injury care and rehabilitation by Sir Ludwig Guttmann at Stoke Mandeville Hospital, south of Oxford, England. Guttmann was a German neurologist and one of two physician brothers who fled Nazi Germany in 1939. The British government, faced with a large number of servicemen with spinal cord injuries, asked Guttmann to set up the National Spinal Injury Center at Stoke Mandeville.

Guttmann developed the principle of early sterile surgical cleaning and removal of debris from a spinal wound. He is also responsible for the method of care of paraplegic patients that is still used today. The methods he established include immobilization of the injured spine until it is healed in order to prevent further damage to the spinal cord; frequently turning the patient to prevent pressure sores; putting a sterile catheter into the bladder every few hours to prevent urinary retention and infection; and training the paralyzed bladder to empty in response to new signals such as pressing on the abdomen. Nurses used enemas to prevent bowel impaction and to train the paralyzed bowel to empty at a regular time each day. Physical therapists moved patients' legs several times a day to reduce the risk of clots forming in the leg veins—a condition called phlebitis. These clots can break loose and travel to the lungs, where they can block the blood flow and kill the patient. Physical therapy is also important to prevent the tendons from tightening up around the knees and hips, reducing the range of motion of the joints (we call this contracture of the joints).

During and after the Second World War, doctors immobilized the injured segment of a spine with a neck brace. More recently, neurosurgeons and orthopedic surgeons have developed internal fixation devices that stabilize the spine. Even with these techniques, patients still need large neck braces for several weeks.

When Guttmann first started treating patients with spinal cord injuries, he had the nurses turn the patients every half hour or so to prevent pressure sores. Later, Homer Stryker, an innovative orthopedic surgeon from Michigan, developed a bed frame that suspends the patient between two layers of canvas covered with sorbo rubber. This frame makes it much easier for the nurses to turn a patient every two hours.

Guttmann and his team paid a good deal of attention to the psychological care of patients. Guttmann trained teams of psychologists and therapists to help the injured servicemen through their early depression. Other veterans who had graduated from Guttman's program provided advice and support. They told new patients about a whole world of possibilities open to them, even if they were paralyzed and bound to a wheelchair.

Guttmann and his team achieved remarkable success. Patient survival improved dramatically, and many patients went on to happy marriages and useful careers in civilian life. The success of the Stoke Mandeville program led to its adoption around the world, the prognosis of spinal cord injury improved globally.

Guttmann believed that playing sports was an important element of rehabilitation. In 1948 he started the Stoke Mandeville Games for paraplegic patients. In 1960, following the Rome Olympics, the Stoke Mandeville Games became the Paralympics, which to this day follow each Olympic Games. (The term *Paralympics* was derived from "parallel Olympics," not from the word *paraplegia*.)

During the Vietnam War, with its new weaponry, many servicemen suffered spinal cord injury from high-velocity bullets. In our cities, similar injuries result from criminal activities and "urban warfare." High-velocity bullets dissipate so much energy as they hit the body that the spinal cord may be damaged irreparably, even if the bullet does not hit the spinal cord itself. Medical technicians deployed with patrols in Vietnam used squeeze bags (called Ambu bags®) to keep alive servicemen with respiratory paralysis from high cervical spine injuries. This sustained patients until helicopters could get them to a ventilator machine at a mobile army service hospital (MASH).

The development of rapid response emergency medical services has resulted in the survival of many people with quadriplegia and respiratory paralysis from high cervical cord injuries. Some are athletes, who are particularly at risk of cervical cord injuries. Marc Buoniconti, son of the professional football player Nick Buoniconti, broke his neck playing college football. With the help of Barth Green and his group in the University of Miami neurosurgery department, Marc was able to survive a high cervical cord injury and now leads a very full and productive life. Later, his father, a guard and linebacker for Notre Dame, the Patriots, and the Miami Dolphins, founded the Miami Project to Cure Paralysis.

Technological advances have continued. For instance, a high spinal cord injury at the level of the fourth cervical vertebra or above stops messages from the respiratory center of the brain from reaching the diaphragm and the muscles that move the ribs when we breathe. Since the phrenic nerves going to the diaphragm remain intact in such patients, surgeons can implant a phrenic nerve stimulator to send impulses to the diaphragm, thus replacing the ventilator.

Researchers have used miniaturization of electronics to develop many new devices in spinal cord research units like the Miami Project to Cure Paralysis. Someone with quadriplegia who is not on a ventilator can control a wheelchair by sucking and blowing on a tube. Marc Buoniconti gets around in this fashion. Either by using this sip and puff technique, or by using any residual movement remaining in a finger, the face, or the neck, people with quadriplegia can use a microswitch to work their phones, computers, doors, and beds.

Servo-assisted "exoskeletons" are frames that fit around the patient and allow him to walk by means of computerized messages and multiple little electrical motors moving the joints. You can imagine how wonderful it is for a paralyzed patient to walk again, even in such a frame. Training on treadmills using these frames can even bring about improvement in muscles and joints.

Psychological counseling and education are important parts of rehabilitation from spinal cord injury for both sexes. Both men and women with spinal cord injury lose the sensation in their sexual organs. For women, pregnancy and childbirth are still possible, however. For both sexes, though the direct pleasure of sexual intercourse is lost in a complete spinal cord injury, other aspects of sexual life can continue. Men with spinal cord injury lose the ability to achieve penile erection but they continue to produce sperm that can be harvested with medical techniques. One of the important advances of spinal cord injury centers is a fertility program that allows men with spinal cord injuries to father children.

It is amazing to look back to the time before the Second World War, when a paraplegic patient had a life expectancy of less than two years. Now, patients in wheelchairs have an almost normal life expectancy and are found in all walks of life. In most developed countries, laws like the Americans with Disabilities Act ensure that patients with spinal cord injury have access to a happy and productive personal and professional life.

Mario was a remarkable young man who overcame all the handicaps that his spinal cord injury and quadriplegia produced. He received treatment in a VA spinal cord rehabilitation unit for twenty months and was released ready to take on the world. He went back to college and started a very successful career in business and finance. He married and adopted a daughter and is active in the National Spinal Cord Injury Association.

## Other Causes of Spinal Cord Damage

Many conditions besides traumatic injuries may cause spinal cord damage. For example, people may develop tumors that compress or infiltrate the spinal cord. A meningioma is one such benign tumor that develops from the dura, the tough covering of the spinal cord. A meningioma grows slowly and may compress the spinal cord over a period of years to produce a slowly worsening paraplegia. A common site of meningioma is the thoracic area. For some reason, women in their middle years of life are more at risk than men.

An ependymoma is a relatively benign tumor of the spinal cord itself. It arises from the cells lining the central canal of the spinal cord and slowly leads to paraplegia or quadriplegia, depending on where it grows in the spinal cord. Often neurosurgeons can totally remove this tumor and prevent it recurring, but the patient may be permanently left with some sensory and motor problems.

Yet another tumor of the spinal cord arises from the astrocytes—cells that support the axons and central nervous tissue. Astrocytomas are malignant and rarely cured by surgery. X-ray therapy can be used to slow their rate of growth.

Blood vessel abnormalities can damage the spinal cord and produce paraplegia or quadriplegia. If a major artery supplying the cord gets blocked—for instance, by atheroma (hardening of the arteries) in the aorta—then the patient suffers a stroke of the spinal cord. In another case, a patient might have been born with a rare abnormal connection between an artery and a vein in the region of the spinal cord. This condition, called an arteriovenous fistula, can either rupture and produce a hemorrhage into the spinal cord or it may suck essential blood away from it. In either situation, the spinal cord is damaged and the patient develops signs of a spinal cord injury.

One of my colleagues, a wonderful surgeon, teacher, and administrator, suffered a different condition that rendered him paraplegic and in a wheelchair for the rest of his life. He suddenly developed what is called transverse myelitis—inflammation across both sides of the spinal cord at a specific point. In only a couple of days, his legs and trunk became numb and he lost the abilities to walk and to move his legs. Imaging studies showed nothing pressing on his spinal cord, and his arteries looked fine. He suffered transverse myelitis before we had MRI scanners, which would have shown an area of the spinal cord swollen with increased watery fluid and damage to the nerve fibers. The lesion in transverse myelitis looks very much like an area of multiple sclerosis; in fact, patients with MS may suffer an episode of transverse myelitis. When this condition develops in a man of fifty or sixty, it is not usually caused by MS, and the patient generally does not improve.

We treat patients with all types of nontraumatic spinal cord damage in the same way as we treat those with traumatic injuries. Fortunately, most nontraumatic conditions cause incomplete spinal cord damage and the patients retain some ability to walk and feel their legs.

## Research to cure spinal cord injury

Research on spinal cord injury in centers like the Miami Project to Cure Paralysis uses laboratory animals to teach us what goes on in injured humans and how to treat them. When given immediately after the injury, high-dose corticosteroids such as prednisone and dexamethasone foster improved recovery in rats. Steroids have not proved to be effective in humans, however. Researchers have discovered other drugs that help the nervous system to withstand injury in animals, but these do not seem to be much use in human spinal cord injury, either.

Axons from both below and above a spinal cord injury begin to regenerate across the injured site. Research has shown that several molecules on astrocytes and other cells inhibit the growth of these regenerating axons. Current research is focused on developing drugs to block the effect of these proteins. Another approach is to introduce stem cells to bridge the gap and perhaps allow the axons to regenerate into the intact spinal cord.

Chapter 9

# The Brain and Cancer

A ndreas was referred to me by a colleague in Greece. He was in his forties and worked as a bank manager in Athens. About six weeks before I saw him, he had noticed difficulty adding up columns of figures. His mathematical skills had always been very strong; that was why he first had become interested in banking. He could not understand why numbers had suddenly become so difficult.

Andreas had gone to my colleague, who had arranged a CT scan of the brain. The scan indicated an ominous mass on the left side of Andreas's brain. My colleague told Andreas that he probably had a brain tumor. He recommended that Andreas go to the United States to benefit from the latest treatment options.

When I examined Andreas, I couldn't find anything wrong with his nervous system, with one exception, arithmetic. He made occasional mistakes adding two-digit numbers and was totally unable to do the more complex calculations of multiplication or division. This was clearly a dramatic change for a person with his background.

I looked at Andreas's brain CT scan from Athens. The plain scan was normal, but the scan taken after he was given intravenous contrast material showed an abnormal area in the temporal and parietal areas of the cerebral cortex, just over his left ear. This is the region that the brain uses for mathematical tasks. A young resident was with me, and he was seeing this CT technique for the first time. I said to him, "Do you see how the contrast-enhanced scan lights up the area where mathematical function is localized in a right-handed man like Andreas? Unfortunately, that looks like a glioma." I used the word *unfortunately* because I knew that this was a bad tumor. Andreas was unlikely to survive for another year.

We arranged for an MRI scan, which is better than CT for showing the extent of the tumor, and I asked my neurosurgical colleague to see Andreas. The MRI scan showed that the tumor was much more extensive than you might expect from his very limited neurological deficit. Gliomas tend to spread tentacles into parts of the brain adjacent to where the tumor first started, well before any signs of neurological damage develop.

My neurosurgical colleague and I sat with Andreas and his wife and explained the situation. We told them Andreas probably had a nasty brain tumor that goes by the Latin name glioblastoma multiforme. We would need to remove a small piece of the tumor through a hole drilled in his skull and look at it under a microscope to be sure about the nature of the tumor. After that, Andreas would probably need X-ray treatment.

Andreas asked me if the tumor could be cured. I said that, if he did in fact have a glioblastoma, then it was rare for the treatment to produce a true cure. Rather, radiation treatment could slow down the tumor's growth and give him a longer period of quality survival. Nevertheless, as I told Andreas and his wife, I have seen two glioblastoma patients who were totally cured. One was an eleven-year-old child who is now in his forties, and the other is an attorney friend and patient, who has no sign of recurrence twelve years after his surgery and radiation treatment. The neurosurgeon added that he had another three patients who had been cured. Andreas's wife asked what was special about those patients, and we had to admit that we had no idea. The neurosurgeon then went on to explain the surgery that he proposed for taking the biopsy of the tumor.

# What Is Brain Cancer?

Brain tumors make up only 2 percent of all cancer cases in the United States. About 100,000 new cases of brain tumors are diagnosed each year, and more than 300,000 Americans currently live with a brain tumor. About 13,000 Americans die of a malignant brain tumor each year. In 2009, it cost an average of about $7000 per month to treat a patient with a malignant brain tumor in the United States. Many brain tumors shorten life, reduce productivity, and impose a major burden on the patient and his family. About 7 percent of brain tumors occur in children.

Metastases from a cancer somewhere else in the body make up about half of all brain tumors. These are called secondary brain tumors. Cancer of the lung, breast, and kidney are common culprits of these secondary tumors. Tumors that arise from intrinsic brain tissue are called primary brain tumors. Among these, benign tumors such as meningiomas and neurofibromas make up 20 percent of intracranial and spinal tumors. Gliomas, which are cancers of the supporting cells of the brain, make up the remaining 30 percent of brain tumors. Malignant gliomas, called glioblastoma multiforme, comprise about half of all gliomas.

Brain cancers are more frequent in older people, and men are affected more than women. For an unknown reason, meningiomas are an exception to this rule, and they affect women more than men. Children have very different tumors from those that occur in adults.

# Types of Brain Tumors and the Tests
# Used in Their Diagnosis

There are many types of brain tumors, and each one behaves differently. It is very important for doctors to be able to determine the exact type of tumor because the prognoses and required treatments differ greatly, depending on the tumor-type. Wherever possible, doctors remove a piece of the tumor to examine under a microscope. This procedure is called a brain biopsy. Some tumors arise in parts of the brain that are so delicate, such as the brain stem, that biopsy is too dangerous. In that case, doctors have to administer treatment based on the likely nature of the tumor, its location, and information from MRI scans.

Specialists called neuropathologists examine the biopsy specimen under a microscope. They use tissue-staining agents to help them identify the tumor type. Some tumors are benign and slow growing, while others, like Andreas's glioblastoma, are very rapidly growing and highly malignant. The tests used to diagnose these different tumors are very similar, but their treatment varies depending on both the type of tumor and the tumor's location in the brain.

CT scans can be performed with or without contrast. Contrast medium is an iodine-containing compound dissolved in saline and administered into the vein of the patient. The iodine shows up well on the CT scan. Normally, the uniquely tight structure of brain blood vessel walls—known as the blood-brain barrier—blocks the entry of the contrast medium into the brain; therefore, in a normal brain scan the contrast material is present only in the blood vessels. A brain tumor, especially a malignant one like a glioblastoma, breaks down the blood-brain barrier and lets the iodine-containing compound get into the tumor mass. This "lights up" the tumor on the CT scan.

MRI scans show brain tumors better than CT scans do because on an MRI scan, tumor tissue looks sharply different from normal brain tissue. A contrast medium called gadolinium can be used to "light up" the tumor. Tumors cause the brain to swell with excess water, which shows up well on MRI scans as well. Different tumors have very different appearances on CT or MRI scans, and a neuroradiologist can usually be fairly certain of her diagnosis of the tumor-type.

The cause of cancer in general is still an enigma. We know that some irritants, called carcinogens, cause specific cancers. For example, cigarette smoke causes lung cancer. We also know that some genes cause cancer to run in families. This is the case with familial breast and colon cancer.

With regard to the nervous system, an inherited disease called neuro-fibromatosis makes the patient vulnerable to several types of tumors of the supporting cells of the brain, spinal cord, and peripheral nerves. If a person's immune system is severely suppressed, especially due to HIV/AIDS, an otherwise benign virus can break out and cause a type of tumor called a primary central nervous system lymphoma. However, we don't know what causes most brain and spinal cord tumors. One theory is that brain cancers are caused by viruses. People have worried that cell phones might cause brain tumors, though this fear seems groundless; brain tumors occurred well before cell phones existed.

Glioblastoma multiforme is the most malignant type of tumor. The cancer spreads rapidly through the brain. Under a microscope many of the cancer cells are bizarre looking, and cells are dividing rapidly to make new daughter cells.

Astrocytoma is less malignant than glioblastoma, meaning that it is slower growing. These tumors are formed from astrocytes, one of the subtypes of supporting brain cells.

Oligodendroglioma is even less malignant than astrocytoma. It is formed from the oligodendroglial cell, another subtype of glia, which forms myelin around the axons in the brain.

Ependymoma is often less malignant than an oligodendroglioma. It is formed from cells that line the insides of the ventricles, the central cavities of the brain, and the spinal cord. This lining is called the ependyma. An ependymoma is particularly found in the cavities of the brain and in the spinal cord.

Meningioma is generally a benign tumor, meaning that it is very slow growing and does not send tentacles of cancer cells to invade the brain, as does a glioblastoma. Rather, it just slowly expands, pressing normal brain out of its way. Meningioma forms from cells of the dura. It usually arises outside the brain but inside the skull.

Medulloblastoma is a very malignant tumor of childhood. It generally occurs in the cerebellum, at the back of the brain.

Pituitary tumors are derived from several types of hormone-secreting cells in the pituitary gland, which lies beneath the center of the brain and just above the nasal cavity. Most of these tumors are benign, but, because they are in a vital area and can only expand upward, they may press on the optic nerves coming from the eyes. This may produce a blind spot. As the tumor enlarges further, it may cause a backup in the flow of CSF from the cavities of the brain. This, in turn, causes a condition called hydrocephalus, literally meaning "water on the brain." Hydrocephalus can cause severe headaches and seriously interfere with brain function.

Some pituitary tumors secrete hormones that produce overactivity of organs such as the thyroid or adrenal glands, or excessive growth of the tissues of the face, hands, and feet in a condition called acromegaly. Some pituitary tumors are very small and picked up only when the patient has an MRI for some other reason. These generally remain embedded in the normal tissue of the gland and are called microadenomas. They cause no symptoms, so doctors simply monitor them with regular MRI scans to make sure that they do not grow.

Craniopharyngioma is a benign cyst that forms in the region of the pituitary gland and slowly expands as fluid accumulates in its cavity. It may produce all the symptoms of a pituitary tumor, except that it does not secrete hormones.

Neurinoma (also called neurofibroma, neurilemoma, and schwannoma) is a tumor that arises from Schwann cells—the peripheral and cranial nerve cells that form myelin sheaths around axons. A neurinoma may also arise from the nerve roots at the base of the brain or in the spinal canal.

An acoustic neurinoma, which causes progressive deafness in one ear, arises from the acoustic nerve that carries hearing messages from the inner ear to the brain. If it gets large enough, it will eventually press on the cerebellum and produce unsteadiness of the limbs (ataxia) on the same side as the tumor. It may press on the sixth cranial nerve and cause difficulty in moving the eye on the same side as the tumor. As the neurinoma enlarges, it presses on the brain stem and causes weakness of the arm and leg on the side opposite from the tumor. A neurinoma on a nerve root in the spine may press on the spinal cord, producing paraparesis or quadriparesis.

Metastasis is a mass of cancer cells that have come from some cancer elsewhere in the body. Metastases are usually very fast-growing tumors that quickly cause symptoms of abnormal brain function. Sometimes a brain metastasis is the first indication that the patient has cancer elsewhere in the body. If a neurologist finds something that looks like a metastasis, he will arrange CT scans of the chest, abdomen, and pelvis, and perhaps a PET scan, to search for this previously silent tumor.

The neurosurgeon took Andreas to the operating room and made a cut in his scalp, all the way down to his skull. He then used a drill similar to one used by a carpenter, but made of stainless steel and carefully sterilized, to bore a hole in Andreas's skull. He put a large, hollow needle through the dura and guided it to the center of the tumor with the aid of a frame attached to the skull and a computer linked to an X-ray machine. This procedure is called a stereotactically-guided brain biopsy. When the needle was in the center of Andreas's tumor, he attached a tube from a suction machine and sucked out a number of specimens for the neuropathologist to examine. As expected, the report came back: "glioblastoma."

## Clinical Features of Brain Tumors

The symptoms produced by a brain tumor vary widely depending on where the tumor is located and how fast it is growing.

If a brain tumor irritates the cerebral cortex, it is likely to produce seizures. These seizures are often focal. They may, for instance, produce Jacksonian epilepsy, where the seizure begins in the hand and corner of the mouth on the side opposite the tumor. If the tumor grows at the back of the brain, either in the cerebellum or in front of the brain stem, it will gradually block the flow of CSF. This will produce hydrocephalus, with gradually worsening headaches that are most troublesome when the patient awakens first thing in the morning. Any type of rapidly expanding tumor within the closed box of the skull may produce early morning headaches due to increased pressure.

Another symptom of a brain tumor is slowly worsening impairment of neurological function. The exact impairment depends on the tumor's location. Andreas was unable to do arithmetic. This symptom indicates damage to the area of the left cerebral hemisphere that processes mathematical thinking.

If the glioma starts deep in the brain or near the part of the cerebral cortex involved in vision, then it may produce loss of vision to the opposite side. If the tumor develops in the front half of the brain and affects the frontal lobes, the patient may experience personality changes and lack of social control.

Another patient might have a tumor growing in the right side of the cerebellum at the back of his brain. Because the cerebellum is the part of the brain where movements of the limbs on the same side are coordinated, this patient would develop slowly worsening incoordination of the right arm and hand. Loss of coordination of the right leg would make the patient tend to veer to the right or simply to fall.

I should mention that all of the above tumors may also occur in the spine. These will compress the spinal cord and produce a slowly increasing paralysis and loss of sensation in the legs, as well as impaired bladder control. The effect of spinal cord tumors is therefore similar to that seen in spinal cord injury, but symptoms of a tumor develop much more slowly. Tumors in the spine tend to produce increasing back pain at the site of the compression.

How fast a tumor is growing influences how rapidly the symptoms develop and progress. Andreas had a fast-growing brain cancer, and his condition advanced rapidly. Within two months, the glioblastoma had spread to other parts of the speech-language centers in his dominant left cerebral hemisphere, and he lost the abilities to read and to understand speech. Later, the tumor caused weakness of his right arm and leg, as well as progressively worsening early-morning headaches. This was what we expected for a glioblastoma. If Andreas's first symptom had occurred five years earlier and his condition had worsened very slowly, then I would have suspected a slow-growing astrocytoma or meningioma.

## Treatment and Prognosis of Brain Tumors

Whether benign or malignant, tumors growing inside the skull may cause death of the patient by pressing on vital structures and raising the intracranial pressure to levels where blood supply to the brain is impeded. Tumors can also interfere with the way that the brain works, and this makes it difficult for the patient to function normally. For all these reasons, brain tumors need to be either removed completely or shrunk to reduce their effects on the brain.

If a neurosurgeon can completely remove the tumor without serious damage to the surrounding brain, then that is the best form of treatment. In many cases, however, the tumor is in such an important area of the brain, or it is so deep, that it cannot be surgically removed. Other tumors infiltrate the brain substance so that it is not possible to remove them surgically. In these cases, treatment is designed to shrink the tumor and slow its rate of growth.

Glioblastomas tend to infiltrate the brain, which means they cannot be removed completely. The type of treatment therefore depends on the tumor's size and location. Andreas's brain cancer was in an area that the neurosurgeon could not touch without taking away Andreas's abilities to speak and to understand language. Though we knew that he would eventually lose those functions because of the spread of the glioblastoma, we did not want to bring on the problems any sooner than necessary. That is why Andreas just had a brain biopsy followed by X-ray treatment to the left side of his brain, rather than a major operation attempting to remove most of the tumor. The radiation was focused on the area of the cancer, as seen on the MRI. In addition, the radiation oncologists radiated the surrounding brain to try to slow the growth of the creeping tentacles of cancer outside the area of the tumor.

Several types of radiation can be used to treat brain tumors. What doctors use depends more on the machines available at a particular medical center than on the nature of the metastasis. The radiation is given in small doses over a prolonged period, often a month, to maximize its effect while reducing side effects. All types of radiation are focused to concentrate the greatest dose to the tumor and the lowest possible dose to the surrounding normal brain.

If Andreas's glioblastoma had been in the frontal lobe of his brain, the neurosurgeon might have done a full-scale operation to remove much of it without producing any loss of function. This procedure is called "debulking." Because of the tentacles of cancer infiltrating Andreas's brain, we knew that it was almost impossible to eliminate the tumor completely, and thus it was impossible to cure him. An alternative treatment, in place of radiation treatment from a machine outside the skull for a patient who had a debulking procedure, would have been for the neurosurgeon to put beads of radioactive material into the walls of the cavity left behind after removal of the glioblastoma. This is called brachytherapy.

Researchers across the world are trying to find better treatments for brain tumors. Intravenous chemotherapy drugs usually do not cross the blood-brain barrier into the brain tissue. Therefore, some experimental protocols call for administering the anticancer drug directly into the artery going to the part of the brain with the cancer, together with a drug that opens up the blood-brain barrier temporarily. Other researchers are modifying viruses that cause encephalitis—inflammatory damage to the brain—to make them target brain cancer cells rather than normal brain cells. Yet other projects involve trying to produce antibodies that attack brain cancer cells.

More benign brain tumors, such as astrocytomas and ependymomas, are better candidates for surgery. Neurosurgeons will try to remove tumors completely, as long as they can do so without causing unacceptable damage to the patient. If the neuropathologist reports that the removed tumor is malignant, the patient usually receives radiation treatment after the surgery. Neurosurgeons can often completely remove meningiomas and neurinomas, and because they are generally benign, the patient will not get radiation treatment. The more benign the tumor, the more likely is neurosurgical removal to be a permanent cure.

If brain scans indicate that a patient has metastases in his brain, then it is obvious that he has a cancer somewhere else in his body, and it probably affects several other organs. Therefore, it will not help him if we subject him to a major neurosurgical operation to take out the brain metastases. His only chance is chemotherapy, often combined with radiotherapy to the brain metastases. Gamma Knife® and CyberKnife® machines are particularly good at aiming the radiation only at the area of each metastasis.

Doctors also must treat the secondary effects of brain tumors. If the tumor causes seizures, doctors use antiepileptic medications to reduce them. Andreas never had a seizure, but the neurosurgeon and I agreed that he should take phenytoin as an "insurance policy" against seizures. The major secondary effect of a brain tumor is that it continues to grow inside the closed box of the skull. This progressively raises the internal pressure to intolerably high levels and produces severe headache. Eventually the patient goes into coma when the intracranial pressure becomes so high that blood flow in the arteries is reduced to dangerously low levels.

Andreas developed raised intracranial pressure three months after he returned to Athens, following his radiation treatment. He started complaining of headaches every morning upon waking up. When my Greek neurologist friend looked at the back of Andreas's eyes with an ophthalmoscope, he could see that there was raised intracranial pressure because the optic disc—where the optic nerve connects with the eye—was swollen. (This is called papilledema.) My colleague knew this meant that the tumor and the edema—the fluid that accumulates around these tumors—had reached a critical volume. He prescribed a high-dose steroid called dexamethasone, which reduces the fluid accumulation in the brain tissue around the tumor.

Andreas's headaches disappeared, but then they came back two weeks later. My colleague increased Andreas's steroid dose several times during the next three months. Eventually, Andreas was taking the maximum dose of steroid but still had headaches that were present most of the time. He also had a very puffy face and high blood pressure because of the side effects of the steroids.

My colleague knew that Andreas was reaching the end of the line. He could have admitted Andreas to the hospital to give him intravenous mannitol, a drug that can reduce edema, but this benefit would have been temporary. By now, Andreas's quality of life was unacceptable, and everyone realized that it was not the time for heroics. He was paralyzed down his right side and could neither speak nor understand anyone. My colleague stopped the steroids and gave Andreas painkillers for the headache. Over the next two days, Andreas gently drifted into a terminal coma. His suffering, and that of his family, ended a few days later.

Andreas's story is the worst example of what can happen with a brain tumor. For many patients the tumor is more benign and does not cause serious problems for months or even years. Some tumors—particularly those that occur in childhood, like medulloblastoma—are often very sensitive to radiation treatment, and they can be cured.

## How Cancers in Other Parts of the Body Affect the Brain

As I described earlier, lung or breast cancer may release cells into the bloodstream. These cells can form metastases that damage the brain or spinal cord. Less commonly, damage to the brain can occur as a result of antibodies against a cancer that is located somewhere other than the brain. The patient's immune system forms these antibodies in an attempt to kill the cancer cells. The antibodies sometimes turn out to be a double-edged sword because they not only kill the cancer cells in an organ like the lung, but they also damage the nervous system. We say that such antibodies are "cross-reacting" with the nervous system cells.

Since another name for cancer is *neoplasm*, the effects of damage to the nervous tissue that results from the remote effects of cancer elsewhere is called a paraneoplastic syndrome. The cancer and the resulting antibodies may develop relatively quickly, and therefore the neurological problem that results from the antibodies may also develop quickly. In a matter of a few months, the patient may become completely disabled as a result of the paraneoplastic neurological damage.

Different cancers, and the different antibodies that form against them, may produce several very different neurological conditions, depending on what part of the nervous system is attacked. Currently, we have little idea why different patients develop these different conditions. The cerebellum is particularly at risk of developing a paraneoplastic cerebellar degeneration, causing the patient to become uncoordinated due to ataxia. He may have slurred speech, difficulty walking and controlling his hands; the picture can look as though he were drunk.

If cancer antibodies attack the sensory neurons of the peripheral nervous system, the patient will develop a sensory neuropathy— damage to the peripheral nerves—producing loss of feeling in the hands and feet, along with difficulty walking that comes about because the patient cannot tell where his feet are without looking at them.

Another rare paraneoplastic condition is limbic encephalitis, in which the antibodies damage the parts of the brain involving memory. The patient also suffers a rapidly developing dementia and often has seizures. Occasionally, the antibodies are directed against the retina, and the patient suffers rapidly deteriorating vision.

Because these neurological conditions are an indirect antibody response to what may be a small and hidden cancer, they are not easy to diagnose. Highly specialized blood tests may pick up some of the antibodies, and MRI scans may show damage to the affected parts of the nervous system. However, the key to diagnosis lies in the neurologist's recognizing that the relatively rapid development of a cerebellar degeneration or a sensory neuropathy is likely to be a paraneoplastic condition, rather than a "simple" degeneration. This recognition leads to a search for the underlying cancer. If one is found, a surgeon may be able to remove it completely and cure the patient of the cancer. The neurological disease might not disappear immediately, however, because the immune system may continue to produce antibodies for months. Eventually the antibodies often disappear, and the neurological disorder improves.

Immunotherapy is an additional treatment for paraneoplastic syndromes. It consists of various approaches to block the effect of the antibodies on the nervous system. Immunotherapy includes high-dose intravenous immunoglobulin (IVIg) that somehow prevents the antibodies from doing their damage; high-dose steroids such as prednisone; and chemotherapy-like drugs such as cyclophosphamide (Cytoxan®) suppresse the lymphocytes that produce the antibodies.

The results of immunotherapy can be quite dramatic, as in the case of Jean, who was sent to me because of a rapidly progressing cerebellar degeneration. At the age of fifty-six, she noticed difficulty with balance and tingling in her feet, followed by slurred speech and loss of fine motor control in her hands. These symptoms gradually worsened; in less than a year she was totally disabled and confined to a wheelchair. She needed help to eat; her speech had become unintelligible.

Despite three very diligent searches during that year, we could not find an underlying cancer, nor could we find any specific antibodies in blood tests. Nevertheless, I still thought it likely that Jean had a paraneoplastic cerebellar degeneration and sensory neuropathy, but I could not prove it, nor could I arrange for a possible culprit tumor to be removed.

I kept Jean well-informed about was happening to her nervous system and why we were doing all the CT and PET scans. She was very disappointed when the tests kept coming back negative. In the end, she asked me, "Is there nothing that you can do for me, doctor?" I told her that we could try immunotherapy, even if we could not find the underlying cancer. I also told her about the risks of immunotherapy. Despite the warnings, she wanted to try. "Doctor, I am totally destroyed," she said. "What have I got to lose?"

Jean had all the complications of high-dose immunotherapy. She lost her hair from the chemotherapy, developed temporary diabetes from the steroids, and got hives as a result of something in the IVIg. However, in three months she was much improved, so we continued the immunotherapy at slightly lower doses for another six months. Eventually she got back to walking with a cane, cooking and taking care of the house, and speaking with only a slight slur. She and I were both delighted.

# Amyotrophic Lateral Sclerosis
## (Lou Gehrig's Disease)

Jim came into my office with his wife, Sara. From the information sheet he had filled in, I saw that he was a forty-year-old lawyer. As we shook hands, I noticed right away that the muscles of his right hand were atrophied. "I've had this twitching of my muscles for a couple of months, and now my right arm is getting weak. Also, I'm not walking well," he said. "Please tell me what's going on." I noticed that Jim's speech was a little slurred, but there was no smell of alcohol on his breath. My heart dropped. I realized that he might have ALS.

I asked Jim more questions about when the speech difficulty had started, whether he had any difficulty swallowing or walking, whether he had any sensory symptoms such as numbness or tingling, and whether there was anyone else in his family who had suffered from a similar condition. I asked Sara whether she had noticed any change in Jim's personality or memory. Then I followed up with a series of questions targeted to find anything in Jim's history that could be responsible for this condition. What illnesses had he suffered? Had he ever had polio? Was he taking any medications, or was he exposed to any poisons that might produce these symptoms?

Then I asked Jim to let me examine him. As he walked into my examination room I saw that he had a stiff-legged gait characteristic of spasticity of the legs. When he undressed, I could see the muscle twitching (fasciculations) that he had mentioned. The muscles of his right hand were wasted, and the muscles of that arm were smaller than they should have been. On the other hand, Jim's reflexes were extremely brisk. He was able to feel a pin prick, a piece of cotton, and the vibration of a tuning fork on every part of his body. His memory was perfectly intact. My suspicion that this was ALS grew stronger.

As gently as possible, I shared my thoughts with Jim and Sara. Sara immediately burst into tears, but Jim seemed remarkably in control of his emotions. He said, "My doctor told me that ALS was one of the conditions that might be causing my symptoms, and Sara and I looked it up on the Internet. We just hoped that you would tell us that it wasn't that."

# What Is ALS?

Americans call ALS "Lou Gehrig's disease" after the famous New York Yankees baseball player of the 1930s. In Spanish it is called ELA (*esclerosis lateral amiotrófica*). In Britain it is known as motor neuron disease (MND), and in France it is *la maladie de Charcot*, after Jean-Martin Charcot, who in 1874 was the first to separate ALS from other chronic neuromuscular diseases and acute poliomyelitis.

ALS is a progressive, degenerative disease of the motor system of the brain and spinal cord. This means that there is progressive sickness and death of both the upper motor neurons, which send their axons down the spinal cord to carry the brain's messages for a limb to move, and the lower motor neurons, which carry the upper motor neurons' commands to the muscles of the face, the tongue, the arms, the trunk, and the legs. The degeneration of these motor neurons occurs very slowly, so that weakness creeps up on the patient.

About 10 percent of ALS patients have someone else in the family who has the disease; they are described as having familial ALS (fALS).

For most patients with fALS, one of the parents and half the siblings are affected by the same disease, and half the patient's children may become affected. This is called dominant inheritance.

The first gene for fALS to be discovered was the gene for superoxide dismutase-1 (SOD-1). This enzyme helps break down superoxide free radicals that may produce oxidative damage to the cell. Loss of the ability to break down free radicals is not the cause of the disease, however. Rather, it seems that the mutant SOD-1 protein poisons the cell. Other genes for fALS are being discovered, and some are related to the movement of materials up and down the long motor nerves in the process called axonal transport, which I describe in Chapter 1.

More than 90 percent of patients with ALS have no family history of the disease and are said to have sporadic ALS (sALS). It seems likely that individuals who develop sALS suffer from the effects of some toxin in the environment that poisons the motor neurons. Many environmental factors have been proposed to cause ALS, including viruses, toxins, vitamin deficiencies, and metabolic abnormalities. Theories of the cause of ALS are numerous; they come and go with each piece of new evidence. Every theory must be viewed with some degree of skepticism until we have the results of further research. I will only describe the theory that I find most exciting at the present time, because it seems intrinsically logical.

In a few isolated areas of the world, ALS has been much more common than elsewhere on the globe. These endemic areas include the island of Guam, the Kii Peninsula of Japan, and Irian Jaya in Indonesia, and in each of these areas the incidence of the disease at its peak was at least one hundred times that in the rest of the world. It has long been hoped that research into the cause of ALS in these endemic areas would reveal the cause of sALS in the rest of the world.

When U.S. troops returned to Guam at the end of World War II, they found that the Chamorro natives had one hundred times more cases of ALS than the rest of the world. Some patients also had Parkinson's disease and dementia. The research of neurotoxicologist Peter Spencer and ethnobotanist Paul Alan Cox has linked the toxic amino acid beta-N-methylamino-L-alanine (BMAA) to ALS cases in Guam.

BMAA is produced by primitive cyanobacteria in the roots of the cycad palm. These cyanobacteria synthesize nutrients for the tree, with BMAA as a side-product. BMAA travels up the cycad palm to its seeds, which the Chamorros use to make flour. The Chamorros also love to eat fruit bats that eat the covering of the cycad palm seeds. The BMAA gets into the brain proteins of the Chamorros and acts as a slow toxin.

Since BMAA-synthesizing cyanobacteria occur worldwide, it is possible that BMAA may be the environmental factor causing ALS. Our research has shown that BMAA is accumulated in the brains of North American patients with both ALS and Alzheimer's disease, but it is not found in normal brains.

Patients with sALS are likely to suffer the effects of the disease because of interplay between the environmental toxin and a genetic predisposition that, in itself, is not strong enough to cause familial ALS. This means that some of the patient's 30,000 genes have minor alterations (polymorphisms) that either make the patient more susceptible to developing the disease or protect the rest of us from getting the disease. If these individuals get a large dose of BMAA, as do the Chamorros of Guam, many will contract the disease. If people are exposed to low concentrations of the toxin, only a small number of people with a genetic susceptibility will get the disease.

Sporadic amyotrophic lateral sclerosis is sometimes said to be rare, but almost one in five hundred of us will die of this disease. When someone is diagnosed with ALS, friends and relatives start talking about it and often find that they or their friends know of several other people who had the disease.

In the United States, about 10,000 new cases are diagnosed each year, and at any one time some 30,000 patients are living with ALS. Men are affected twice as frequently as women, though after menopause women are affected almost as often as men. The disease is rare below the age of twenty, though I had a patient who was fifteen when I made the diagnosis. ALS is most frequent in the sixty- to seventy-year-old age group. Doctors often miss the diagnosis in very elderly patients, because they are just thought to be suffering from old age.

# Tests Used in the Diagnosis of ALS

"How can you be so sure it *is* ALS?" Sara asked. I explained as kindly as possible, "The diagnosis is made on the basis of the history that Jim gave me and the clinical examination that I just did. Jim's muscles are wasting due to degeneration of the lower motor neurons in his spinal cord. He also has brisk reflexes and spastic legs, which are due to degeneration of the upper motor neurons of the brain. He told me that the condition is slowly worsening. Sadly, there is very little else that can produce these changes other than ALS."

Sara asked, "What about all those blood tests, MRIs, electrical tests, and fluid they collected through the needle in the back (spinal tap) that the doctor did on Jim? He told us that they didn't show anything." I explained, "Those were done to make sure that there was nothing else going on in Jim's nervous system that might have caused the symptoms." As in Jim's case, patients are often referred to me when the tests to rule out more common ailments have been completed.

No specific test can diagnose ALS. If the patient is in a family with a gene mutation causing ALS, it may be possible to find that mutation and test a relative who has symptoms and signs of ALS and prove that they have the disease. About 20 percent of patients with fALS have mutations for the gene called SOD1, and commercial DNA tests are available for this gene. DNA tests are not available for most of the other currently known gene mutations, however.

For patients with sALS, the diagnosis is based on the characteristic clinical picture of only upper and lower motor neuron degeneration, as well as the typical progression of the weakness, without any evidence of involvement of any other part of the nervous system. Many patients require a number of tests to rule out any other conditions that might theoretically produce a similar clinical picture. MRI scans of the brain and spinal cord can rule out strokes, tumors, and pressure of intervertebral discs.

Medical personnel also often perform an electric test of the nerves and muscles, called electromyography (EMG), and nerve conduction velocity (NCV) studies. EMG involves putting a thin recording electrode into the muscles of the arms and legs to show the presence of denervation, or degeneration of the lower motor neurons. NCV studies, which involve giving little electric shocks to individual nerves, can detect a condition called multifocal motor neuropathy that can mimic ALS.

Blood tests for signs of inflammation, deficiency of vitamin B12, heavy metal intoxication, and abnormality of thyroid function are often carried out, because all of these conditions occasionally produce neurological conditions that resemble ALS. If a neurologist suspects a disease other than ALS, he may order additional tests that can prove the existence of that other disease.

Sara asked about the spinal tap that Jim's first neurologist had done. As I have mentioned, this test removes a sample of CSF from the small of the back. The CSF of ALS patients, as in Jim's case, is typically normal, so any abnormality suggests that some other disease may be causing the patient's problems.

Let me say something about the diagnosis of ALS and the breaking of bad news to the patient. An experienced neurologist can often make the diagnosis of ALS upon the first examination, but many neurologists dislike informing the patient until it has become absolutely obvious that the disease is ALS. Commonly this reluctance results in a delay of a year or more between the first symptoms and the time when the patient is informed that they have ALS. This delay is very distressing to the patient and family because they are left hanging. The patient does not know what is making him progressively more disabled, and is frustrated that the neurologist keeps doing more and more tests. Often patients come to me after diagnosing themselves based on information on the Internet. Rather than letting patients live in fear, I prefer to tell them at the end of the first consultation what disease seems likely to be the cause of their symptoms, as I did with Jim and Sara.

Sadly, patients with ALS do not always get the most compassionate treatment. Neurologists may make the diagnosis but not inform the patient about ALS with all the compassion that is needed. Probably the doctor feels inadequate, knowing that he has no ability to cure the disease. Patients frequently tell me that their first neurologists said something like this: "You have ALS. It is a fatal, incurable neurological disease, and you are going to die in a year. There is nothing I can do for you, and there is no point in your coming back to see me. Go home, put your affairs in order, and prepare to die." To me, this is completely unacceptable.

Though it is important to give the patient the likely diagnosis as soon as possible, it is also crucial to give him hope when revealing the bad news. As in the case of Jim and Sara, I always say that I will be with them throughout the course of this illness. I will provide them with treatment, knowledge about how to deal with the effects of the disease, and hope that we can do something to cure it.

## The Clinical Features of ALS

ALS is very variable in its presentation and progress. It can begin as slurring of speech and difficulty in swallowing. It can begin in one arm or one leg. It can even present with shortness of breath. It can start in the upper motor neurons and cause spasticity (stiffness of the limbs), which is shown by slowness of voluntary movement of the limbs. Spasticity is accompanied by excessive briskness of the tendon reflexes, as measured by tapping a tendon with a small, rubber-tipped hammer. Normally there is a small jump of the leg upon the hammer's impact, but if someone has upper motor neuron damage, the leg will jerk up violently. Degeneration of the lower motor neurons causes fasciculations and muscle atrophy.

Characteristically, ALS starts in one part of the body and gradually spreads. Thus, it may start in one arm and spread down to the leg on the same side, then across to the other arm. It may start in the leg, the arm, the mouth and throat, or the muscles involved in breathing.

The disease's rate of progression also differs from one patient to another. If difficulty with breathing or swallowing appears early, the patient may only live for a few more months. The average survival of ALS patients is about three to five years. However, about 10 percent of patients live for ten years. In some patients the disease appears to reach a plateau. Famed physicist Stephen Hawking is an example of someone with very slowly progressive ALS. He has had an exceptionally productive life despite his disability.

There are a few rare conditions that may be misdiagnosed as ALS. They are termed ALS mimics. Most of these conditions involve only lower motor neuron damage, and some of them are treatable. It is therefore very important that the neurologist make sure patients are not suffering from one of these conditions, such as multifocal motor neuropathy, which is treatable.

## Treatment and Prognosis of ALS

Unfortunately, we have only one drug that has been shown to affect the progress of ALS. It is called riluzole (Rilutek®), and it slows down the disease by about 25 percent. At present we have no way to halt the condition or to cure it. Riluzole has its cons, including high cost, occasional side effects, and limited benefits.

I believe in being as honest as possible with my patients. I tell them that if I had ALS and could afford riluzole, there is no doubt I would take it. However, if I did not have health insurance and needed to "sell the farm" to get the drug, I would not make the sacrifice to gain the relatively small benefit. An individual patient cannot tell that the drug is doing anything. It does not arrest or improve the symptoms, and its benefit can only be detected through trials involving many patients.

Jim was fortunate enough to have health insurance that would pay 95 percent of the total cost of riluzole, which is nearly $9,000 per year. I gave Jim a prescription for one 50-milligram tablet twice a day on an empty stomach. I also arranged for him to get monthly blood tests, since riluzole can irritate the liver.

Researchers have carried out scientific trials of more than fifty other potentially effective drugs for ALS over the last thirty years. These studies are called double-blind placebo-controlled trials, in which one group of patients is randomly allocated to take the active drug and another group is assigned to take a placebo (a sugar pill that looks identical to the active drug). Neither the patient nor the testing doctors knows which patient is getting which preparation until the code is broken at the end of the trial. None of tested drugs have been effective, and a few actually worsened the disease. Nevertheless, therapeutic trials are important, not only because they offer the prospect of finding an effective medication for ALS, but also because they give patients and their families hope.

Only when we know the cause of ALS, will we be able to treat it. For instance, in those patients where we know they have a mutation of SOD1, researchers are planning treatment trials to block the synthesis of this protein. And if the BMAA theory is correct, we will be able to design treatments that will either prevent the toxin from getting into the brain or flush it out of the body.

Most patients never give up the belief that there is a cure for ALS out there *somewhere*. This makes them vulnerable to charlatans offering everything from stem cell therapy and chelation to whatever is the latest fad. On the Internet, self-proclaimed cures of ALS (and many other diseases) tout testimony from individuals who have obtained what is usually described as "remarkable improvement." None of these "cures" have ever been substantiated by further research. Each so-called cure costs the patient and his family a great deal of money because doctors know that there is no evidence that the drug works. Patients are simply paying the modern version of a snake oil salesman.

ALS is perhaps the most terrible of the neurological degenerations for the patient, and it is the most difficult for the neurologist. We know that everyone has to die; we simply do not want to watch it happening. Books have been written about the remarkable philosophical attitude that many ALS patients develop as they suffer progressively more disability. The strength of the human spirit in the face of ALS is amazing to behold.

The prognosis of ALS is not always as bleak as the Internet indicates, however. Younger patients tend to live longer than those who are over the age of sixty. Half of patients with ALS live for more than five years after their diagnosis, and some live longer than fifteen years. Most people, like Jim and Sara, believe that ALS is a certain death sentence. Though this is usually the eventual outcome, it is not invariably so. I have seen five ALS patients recover from the condition. I had to tell one of them that I could no longer sign his forms for continuing disability payments because he had improved so much. He was quite angry.

Jim and Sara came back to see me about a week after our initial consultation so that I could answer the many questions that had inevitably arisen after they left my office the first time. Jim's first new question was, "What stage am I at with my ALS?" He had read on the Internet that people with ALS go through stages, and they have only so long to live when they reach each of the stages. I replied, "There really are no stages, nor can I tell you how long you have to live; that's what you really are asking. Different patients progress at very different rates. Some patients die in six months, and others live ten years or more." I told Jim I'd try my best to answer his question about prognosis in another three months, by which time I could measure his ALS's speed of progression.

Since we cannot cure ALS at present, it is important that we help the patient to maintain the highest quality of life. There is a worldwide network of neurologists and multidisciplinary clinics specializing in ALS. These specialized clinics care for patients and help them maintain quality of life, while also trying to find the cause of and cure for the disease. In the United States and Canada, these ALS centers can be found by accessing the Web sites of the Muscular Dystrophy Association (www.mdausa.org) and the ALS Association (www.alsa.org). There are similar organizations in many other developed countries around the globe.

Patients with ALS are faced with the worst thing they have ever known. They need the support of a caring neurologist who is knowledgeable about ALS. They need professional help, information, and support as their ALS progresses. At multidisciplinary clinics they can receive the services of physical, occupational, speech, and respiratory therapists, as well as psychological help, wheelchairs, hoists, home adaptations, and respiratory assistance. The ALS clinics can help patients and their families navigate the health care bureaucracy. Not every patient with ALS is fortunate to live in a part of the country with a multidisciplinary ALS clinic, but in Jim's case I was able to offer him the services of my own.

Jim lost 10 pounds in the three months after our first visit because he was having difficulty swallowing. I said, "Jim, if you are losing weight, then you are starving your motor neurons and they are going to die sooner. Good nutrition can prevent the disease from accelerating. What you need is a gastrostomy tube."

Jim had read about this, and he was totally opposed to the idea. "I would rather die than have one of those things!" he said.

"It's not terrible," I assured him. "You're put to sleep with a little general anesthetic, the tube is put through your belly wall into your stomach, and you wake up a few minutes later. The place on your belly where the tube goes in may be a little sore for a couple of days, but after that it is completely painless. You can cover it and do anything you want—bathe, swim, have sex … anything!"

Jim and Sara left to consider this and came back a month later. By this time Jim had lost another six pounds and he accepted the gastrostomy tube. Two months later, through tube feeding, he had put on 12 pounds and was feeling much less fatigued.

Difficulty with speech and swallowing can be caused by degeneration of the lower motor neurons that lie in the bulbar region of the brain stem. This produces paralysis (palsy) of the muscles of the face, tongue, and throat. Hence, the paralysis is called bulbar palsy. Difficulty with speech and swallowing can also be caused by damage to the upper motor neurons that *control* the lower motor neurons of the bulbar region. Damage to these upper motor neurons produces a condition called pseudobulbar palsy. The prefix *pseudo* does not imply that the condition is false. It simply means that the condition looks somewhat like the lower motor neuron type of bulbar palsy, but it is actually caused by upper motor neuron problems.

Difficulty with swallowing saliva causes embarrassing drooling called sialorrhea. This can be treated with medications that inhibit the secretion of saliva, such as atropine, amitriptyline (Elavil®), and glyco-pyrrolate (Robinul®). Injections of botulinum toxin (Botox®) into the salivary glands can also cut down saliva production.

Depression is an inevitable effect of ALS that can be effectively treated with antidepressant medications like amitriptyline (Elavil®), sertraline (Zoloft®), or duloxetine (Cymbalta®). Sometimes, the care-giver needs antidepressant medications as much as the patient does. Psychological counseling for both the patient and the caregiver is often helpful.

At one of his clinic visits, Jim burst into a flood of tears and sobbed uncontrollably when I asked him how he and Sara were handling the stress. He was suffering from what I call emotional incontinence. Jim was unable to control his emotions, just as someone with urinary incontinence is unable to control his bladder. Many patients have told me that it is not depression that causes these episodes of uncontrollable crying; they simply cannot control their emotions, and it embarrasses them. Understandably, caregivers find it difficult not to react as though the patient were desperately depressed, and it is helpful when I tell them that the patient is truly not sad. Emotional incontinence can be suppressed with antidepressant medications.

Jim and Sara came to see me urgently three months later because Jim had choked during the previous night and had difficulty catching his breath. We measured the maximum amount of breath that he could take in and then blow out of his lungs (this is called forced vital capacity), which is about three to four liters in a normal individual. Jim's forced vital capacity was 40 percent of normal. It was time to discuss respi-ratory support with him and Sara. I said, "Jim, your breathing is now becoming affected by the ALS. With a forced vital capacity of 40 percent, at night, when the breathing is naturally shallower, you are becoming short of oxygen in your blood. That's dangerous because it makes the disease progress faster. I can give you an apparatus called a BiPAP [bilevel positive airway pressure], which pushes air through your nostrils into your lungs to assist your breathing at night. It's not the ventilator and the hole in your windpipe that you fear so much."

I showed Jim a model of a human head with the nosepiece and BiPAP attached. I explained, "At the beginning it may be difficult to get used to sleeping with this on your face and with the machine wheezing by your bedside. However, most people eventually tolerate it and find that they are much less tired during the day." Jim agreed to use it, and in two days the life support company arrived at his house with the machine. He found that the BiPAP was a great help.

Jim's condition progressed more rapidly than I had hoped. Within eighteen months of the diagnosis, he was confined to a wheelchair. Sara had to do everything for him, including feeding him through the gastrostomy tube, putting on the BiPAP, bathing him, and helping him go to the bathroom. As she said, Jim had become just like a baby. He couldn't speak, but he could communicate with Sara through a letter board by nodding and shaking his head.

In our early consultations, Jim had discussed end-of-life issues with Sara and me. He had made sure we understood what to do if his breathing should fail: "I do not want to be brought back from the grave," he said. "Just let me die peacefully, without suffering."

Jim had signed three important documents. The first was his living will. He had used the standard form but had had added that he wanted to donate his organs after he died. The second document was the health care surrogate form, by which he appointed Sara to make all the medical decisions and to sign all the papers if he became totally incapacitated, unable to communicate, or unconscious. The third document was the durable power of attorney, which appointed someone whom he designated (Sara, in this case) to sign all legal papers if he became totally incapacitated or unconscious.

It was now time for me to talk about hospice care. I went to see Jim and Sara at their home because it was so difficult for her to get him into the car and come to the clinic. I said, "Jim, I recommend that I arrange for hospice services to assist Sara in looking after you. Your breathing is getting pretty limited. Some night you could get into the situation where you're fighting for every breath, and Sara is going to be terrified. Jim, unless we get you hospice services, if this happens, Sara will have no alternative but to call 911. You will be rushed to the nearest hospital, and you will wake up to find yourself on a ventilator with a tube in your throat."

Jim nodded to indicate he understood.

I continued, "The hospice nurses and physician will be available to you and Sara 24/7. If you are getting to the terminal stage, they will come at any hour of the night or day to give you sedatives, oxygen, and morphine. These will take away your distress and hunger for air, and you will be able to die peacefully in your sleep." By now, Jim and Sara were in tears and I wasn't much better. However, they both knew that this was what Jim wanted.

A couple of days later the hospice staff started to provide home services. Jim lasted another eight months, with increasing help from hospice services, the BiPAP, oxygen, and the gastrostomy tube. Then one night he simply drifted off to sleep and did not wake in the morning. Sara told me that she felt it was a blessed relief for Jim to be finished with his suffering, but that she felt guilty about thinking that way. I reminded her that Jim himself had made the decision that he did not want to go onto a ventilator, and she was comforted by this thought.

The medical care situation of many countries is different from that in the United States and Europe. In Japan, for instance, when respiratory failure appears, the patient receives a tracheotomy and ventilator, and the health system provides services to allow the patient to remain at home on the ventilator. In other countries, respiratory support is never provided for patients with ALS.

# Other Motor Neuron Diseases

A small number of patients have an autoimmune disease in which the body produces antibodies against its own motor neurons. Anti-immune therapy can control this disease, which is called multifocal motor neuropathy and is one of the ALS mimics.

There are many other motor neuron diseases. One example, infantile spinal muscular atrophy (or Werdnig-Hoffmann disease), affects infants and produces progressive paralysis of all muscles and death by two years of age. Hereditary spastic paraplegia comes on in juvenile or adult years, and produces progressive stiffness of the legs and brisk reflexes, that may put the patient in a wheelchair within ten years. These conditions do not look anything like ALS. In addition, a number of adult patients who have pure upper motor neuron degeneration are said to have primary lateral sclerosis. Others have pure lower motor neuron degeneration and are described as having progressive muscular atrophy. These conditions occur in adults and progress in a rather similar fashion to ALS, though they may be slower. Many neurologists think that they are therefore just subtypes of ALS.

## Chapter 11

# Migraine and Other Headaches

Almost everyone has occasional headaches, and there are many types and causes. An experienced neurologist can relatively easily separate the different types on the basis of a patient's description, and often no laboratory tests are needed to make the diagnosis. In fact, making the diagnosis of migraine, the commonest cause of recurrent headaches, requires only the quintessential history-taking skill of the neurologist. This is because laboratory tests provide no help, other than to rule out a tumor or some of the other uncommon causes of head pain.

## Clinical Features of Migraine

Migraine is a chronic condition in which the patient suffers from repeated attacks of headache. The nature of the pain is most often throbbing and centered over the forehead and eyes, the temples, or the back of the head. At times, only half the head is affected by pain.

Migraine attacks may last from half an hour to several days. Often patients experience what we call an aura—something that precedes the pain and tells the patient she is going to get a headache in a few minutes. The aura is frequently a bright spot in front of the eyes or a blurring of vision. The patient often feels nauseated, and lights and noise seem almost painful. Headaches return with varying frequency from daily to only once every few years. Migraine has many other manifestations, as I will discuss shortly.

Migraine is the most common cause of recurrent headaches, though people often mischaracterize them as sinus headaches because they believe that migraine headaches must be excruciatingly painful. That is not always the case; in fact, migraine attacks can come without any headache. These attacks are sometimes called migraine sine migraine or acephalgic (meaning "no headache") migraine. Neurologists sometimes use the term *migraineur*, which was borrowed from the French to describe patients with migraine syndromes of all types.

Reports on the incidence of chronic recurrent migraine headaches vary considerably. One estimate is that migraine affects 20 percent of women and 7 percent of men in developed countries, but I believe this is a gross underestimate. Many women do not realize that the headaches that they get at the time of their periods are migraine. Door-to-door surveys indicate that 60 percent of women and 25 percent of men have at least occasional recurrent headaches. Migraine seems to occur in certain personality types, particularly those who are anxious, obsessive, and hardworking, and it is more common in people with epilepsy.

Migraine characteristically begins in a patient's teenage years, though it may appear for the first time in the elderly or in young children. In the United States, at least 30 million people suffer from chronic migraine, and at least two-thirds of them have two or more severe headaches a month. Some of the headaches are severe enough to make the patient stay home from work, or to be less productive than normal while staying at work. The average severe migraineur loses two to four work days per year because of headaches. Several estimates suggest that migraine costs the United States more than $15 billion per year.

For some migraine sufferers, the headaches are totally unbearable. I have seen grown men bang their heads against the wall with one of the variants of migraine, called periodic migrainous neuralgia or cluster headaches. In the total scheme of things headaches may be relatively unimportant compared with stroke, cancer, or ALS, but frequent headaches severely reduce the quality of life for the sufferer.

## Classification of migraine

People who have visual auras before the beginning of a migraine headache are said to suffer from classical migraine. They make up about one-third of patients with migraine. Two-thirds of patients have recurrent migraine-type headaches without visual auras, and they are said to have common migraine. Additional types of migraine include cluster headaches, hemiplegic migraine, ophthalmoplegic migraine, and acephalgic migraine; I will discuss these shortly.

## Clinical features of classical and common migraine

Patients with classical migraine get a visual warning before the headache begins. Typically this starts as a bright spot in front of both eyes, just at the point of focus. I am a migraineur myself and have had this many times. At first I usually misinterpret it. I think to myself, "I need to get my glasses changed. I can't read the fine print." Then I realize that the bright spot is spreading out and becoming a bright zigzag as though I am looking through water and that this means that I am having another migrainous aura.

The aura's area of distortion usually affects just one half of the visual field. The wavy area gradually spreads outward from the center, and at the same time my central vision clears, allowing me to read again. Migrainous auras may occur without an accompanying headache, which is frequently the case for me. For most people, however, fifteen minutes to two hours later they start to feel a throbbing headache, commonly on one side of the head. The reason for the throbbing is that the arteries of the scalp are swollen and tender during the migraine attack, and each pulse of blood pressure in them produces a throb of pain. No one knows why migraine headaches characteristically affect one side of the head, but this feature gave rise to the term historical term *"hemicrania,"* which eventually became contracted to *migraine.*

Although an ache in half the patient's head may lead to a diagnosis of migraine, frequently migraine headaches are felt across the brow, in both temples, or at the back of the head and neck. Usually patients complain that light bothers their eyes, (this is called photophobia) and that loud noises are painful (phonophobia). Patients often feel nausea, and some migraineurs will get no relief for their headache until they vomit. The headache may last for hours or even days, and often patients need to "sleep it off" in a dark room until the pain passes.

Migraine sufferers often have recurrent nausea and vomiting in childhood without headaches. A child in this situation is said to have acephalgic migraine, or cyclical vomiting, and will most likely go on to have typical migraine headaches when they grow up. When I was a child my family doctor told my mother that I was suffering from acidosis (a condition no longer to be found in medical textbooks), and I used to think I had a recurrent upset stomach because I did not want to go to school (school phobia). Only after I became a neurologist did I realize that school wasn't the problem—it was the fact that I had migraine.

Many people have a strong history of migraine in their family; often one of their parents and grandparents, as well as several siblings and children, have the condition. At the age of two and a half, my eldest son said, "Daddy, half my head hurts," and I knew that he had inherited my migraine. Several genes have been discovered to be responsible for dominantly inherited migraine.

For unknown reasons, in the years before puberty, migraine tends to occur more frequently in boys than girls, but after puberty it is more common in females because of the hormonal changes associated with the menstrual cycle. Headaches in women often occur in the premenstrual phase of their cycle.

Migraine headaches are often precipitated by stress, though occasionally people have what is called relaxation migraine because the headaches come when stress is relieved. I had a wonderful editorial assistant who kept all of my journal work efficiently organized. She was prostrated most Saturdays by a severe relaxation migraine headache. We do not understand exactly how stress and migraine attacks are interrelated, but migraineurs well know that the connection exists.

Some migraine sufferers find that certain foods, such as cheese, chocolate, red wine, or spicy foods, may bring on an attack of migraine. Humid weather and strong perfumes can do the same. Many of the food items that precipitate migraine attacks contain chemicals called amines, such as tyramine, that make blood vessels constrict or dilate. How strong odors and changes in barometric pressure produce an attack is not known.

People often find that they can relieve their migraine headaches with caffeine. The reason is not fully understood. Caffeine stimulates receptors on neurons and blood vessels, which probably explains how it works. Many people find that withdrawal from caffeine precipitates a severe migraine attack.

The frequency of migraine attacks varies greatly from person to person. Some people have a migraine only once or twice in their lives, while others have several terrible attacks each week. The headaches' severity also varies greatly. For some patients the headache is very mild, and two aspirin tablets are enough provide relief. Others have to go to the nearest hospital emergency department because the pain is so severe that they need an injection of a narcotic painkiller. As of now, we do not know why the experience of migraine varies so dramatically from one person to the next.

Patients with migraine frequently feel weird during an attack and are aware of being mentally slowed. This is probably due to reduced cerebral blood flow during the migraine attack.

Migraine is one of the causes of a fascinating condition called transient global amnesia (TGA). I was sitting at my desk one day putting together a talk for a visit to another medical school when I was suddenly unsure of what I was doing. I knew that I was selecting slides, but I was not sure why. A few minutes later, I even became confused about why I was sitting at the desk. The confusion was patchy, however, because at that same moment I thought to myself, "I must be having a TGA. Well, that's interesting! I'd better sit back and enjoy it!" The confusion went on for about ten minutes, and then my mind gradually began to clear; I started to remember the upcoming academic visit and why I was sitting at my desk. About fifteen minutes later, I developed a mild headache and some nausea. It was only then that I realized that my TGA was caused by migraine. The reason for this experience was probably reduction of the blood supply or electrical inhibition of the memory areas of the brain. Both of these phenomena occur as part of a migraine attack.

## Complicated migraine

Not infrequently, patients with migraine have some neurological symptoms in addition to the visual auras, headache, nausea, and vomiting. Many will complain that their scalp is tender or numb on the side of the headache. More rarely an arm or a leg goes numb and weak (this symptom is associated with hemiplegic migraine). Others may have double vision due to weakness of some of the muscles moving the eye; this condition is called ophthalmoplegic migraine. Cases in which there is both headache and some other significant neurological dysfunction are said to be "complicated migraine" and the neurological symptoms resolve within an hour or two. Sometimes these forms of complicated migraine run in families and are due to genes that are different from those responsible for the more common forms of familial migraine.

When patients have the first attack of complicated migraine, many are convinced they are having a stroke. Although this is not usually the case, very rarely migraine may cause a stroke. Stroke-like symptoms and signs may be caused by spasms of blood vessels of the brain during the migraine attack. Therefore, patients with complicated migraine should not be given drugs like ergotamine or sumatriptan (Imitrex®), which tend to constrict the cerebral arteries. However, it is equally likely that the neurological problems in complicated migraine result from electrical inhibition of the neurons. I will say more about this in the section on the cause of migraine.

## Cluster headaches

Cluster headaches are just what the name implies: the headaches come in clusters. An individual headache is usually brief, lasting five minutes to an hour, and it generally comes once a day. A cluster of daily headaches appears without reason, may last for weeks or months, and then disappears as mysteriously as it began, only to return one or two years later. The pain frequently affects just one eye, which becomes red and teary. The nose on that side often becomes blocked, and the forehead on the side of the pain may sweat.

Because cluster headache pain is more like the shooting nerve pain associated with trigeminal neuralgia, the condition is often called periodic migrainous neuralgia. For an unknown reason, men are five to ten times more likely to get cluster headaches than women, and the onset is usually between the ages of thirty and fifty. The pain can be so severe that some patients have committed suicide to escape the daily recurrence of unbearable pain.

## Tests that are done on patients with migraine

If a neurologist hears a typical history of migraine from a patient, he will not usually do any complex investigation, such as an MRI. Migraine is so rarely caused by an underlying problem with the brain's blood vessels, such as an aneurysm or arteriovenous malformation, that brain scans are rarely justified. I occasionally do an MRI to relieve the patient's anxiety that he has a tumor or aneurysm, since this stress may cause a vicious cycle leading to worsening of his recurrent migraine headaches. But I do tell patients that the MRI is to relieve *their* anxiety, not mine. We used to think that imaging studies were required if the headache was always restricted to one side, but we now know that there is no increased risk of an underlying blood vessel problem in this situation.

However, it can be difficult to diagnose migraine if the patient is not a good historian, or if the attacks are unusual. For instance, a colleague recently sent me a young lady with the strange complaint of a cold pressing sensation coming from the top of her head and down one side of her face. This happened every month and terrified her. She had no pain, and therefore my colleague did not consider migraine. However, when I found that these episodes occurred at the time of her menstrual periods, that she lost her appetite when they arrived, and that she needed to go into a dark room because the light bothered her during the attack, it was clear that she had migraine without headache. Her attacks disappeared after she started taking antimigraine medication for five days at a time during her periods.

## Cause of migraine

Humans have suffered from migraine headaches since earliest recorded times. The writings of the ancient Egyptians, Greeks, and Romans contain references to hemicrania (pain on one side of the head). Thomas Willis, the great English anatomist and physician of the seventeenth century, concluded that migraine was caused by enlargement of the blood vessels inside the head. In his 1873 treatise *On megrim, sick headache, and some allied disorders: A contribution to the pathology of nervestorms*, Edward Liveing suggested that the relationship between migraine and epilepsy was so strong that both were caused by "nervestorms"— increased electrical activity of the brain. Recent research has shown that he was partly right.

There are two main theories about what causes migraine: the vascular theory and the neuronal theory. In the neurological literature, the pendulum of popularity has swung back and forth between these two theories for the last fifty years. A patient experiencing a migraine attack often has swollen temporal arteries and pallor of the face on the side of the headache. PET scans show increased cerebral blood flow

225

when the patient is in the midst of the headache phase, but during the aura phase blood flow may be decreased. These facts support the vascular theory of migraine.

Support of the neuronal theory includes the fact that migraine may be initiated by the same stimuli that may precipitate epileptic seizures— stress, sleep deprivation, and psychedelic modern paintings. Moreover, the zigzag lines of a visual aura are caused by a wave of impairment (inhibition) of the activity of the neurons of the visual cortex.

I think it is likely that both the vascular and the neuronal theories are true. Certainly, medicines associated with either theory may be effective in controlling migraine headaches.

In two rare conditions, migraine is just one of the symptoms of a more complex neurological disease. Both diseases may cause strokes, and both are caused by genetic mutations. The first disease has a long medical title that is shortened to MELAS, and it is caused by a mutation of the DNA of mitochondria. The other disease goes by an equally long name that gave rise to the acronym CADASIL, and it is caused by a mutation of a gene in the nuclear DNA. Researchers are still trying to find out how these mutations cause strokes and migraine, and more important, how to treat these diseases.

## Treatment of migraine

The first treatment for migraine is to prevent the headaches in the first place. When I see a patient for the first time, I start by determining what factors precipitate the migraine attack and then develop strategies to avoid these precipitants. Cutting out foods that tend to cause migraine attacks, such as cheese and red wine, may reduce the frequency and severity of the headaches. If migraines are associated with menstrual periods, antimigraine medications started three days before the period and continued for the first two days of the period will usually prevent the headaches. If the headaches are particularly associated with stress, relaxation therapy and medicines that relieve tension may help.

If migraine headaches happen more than two or three times a month, and if the patient is prostrated by pain, she will need preventive treatment. Medications that prevent migraine attacks fall into three main classes. The first is the antidepressant class of drugs. Antidepressants work in several ways: they help alleviate some of the underlying stress that precipitates the migraine; they raise the pain threshold; and they block the neurotransmitters responsible for the neuronal aspects of migraine.

The second group of medications works on the vascular system by blocking the reactivity of the brain's arteries. The main categories of these drugs are calcium channel blockers and beta blockers, both of which are also used for treating hypertension and angina. Both categories of drugs tend to lower the blood pressure and cause dizziness and faint feelings. The beta blockers may also cause depression, exacerbate asthma, and block the ability of the heart rate to increase when a patient exercises.

The third group of antimigraine medications is antiepileptic drugs. Several have proved to be effective in suppressing migraine headaches. I usually start with valproate (Depakote®), except in the cases of young children, for whom the drug carries a risk of damaging the liver. Other neurologists use topiramate (Topamax®) to prevent migraine attacks.

I have treated a fascinating family that suffers from not only migraine but also severe muscle pains. The oldest daughter, Becky, was twelve when she was referred to me because of these muscle pains. Her school performance had deteriorated badly; she was missing four out of five days at school because of the pains. They had started around the age of six and had gradually worsened. They were particularly bad when she exercised, but her muscles also hurt even at rest. I learned that Becky also had quite frequent migraine headaches, as did her mother and several of her siblings, and I picked up that the muscle pains were much worse whenever she had a headache. Migraines came almost every day. On the few days when she was headache-free, she had no problems with her muscles and went to school.

Though Becky was a somewhat withdrawn teenager, I did not think that she was suffering from school phobia. I had no idea what was causing the muscle pains and have never seen migraine to cause this symptom. Nevertheless, it seemed that the headaches were too good a clue to miss. I treated her with verapamil, a calcium channel blocker, on the remote chance that the muscle pains were related to spasm of the blood vessels supplying the muscles. If nothing else, I thought, the treatment might help her migraine.

The verapamil reduced the frequency of Becky's headaches to one a month, and her muscle pains largely disappeared. Over the next three years the headaches and muscle pains reappeared at times as she grew, and she needed a higher dose of verapamil. Over the years I added her brother, two sisters, and mother to my list of patients, since they all had migraine and, to varying extent, muscle pains. For all of them verapamil has been the wonder drug, while beta blockers, valproate, and antidepressants have been completely ineffective. I assume that this family has a mutation of a gene that relates to the control of blood vessels in the brain and the muscles.

After prevention, the second important part of treating migraine is to suppress the individual headache. For many patients the headache is not bad, and simple painkillers like aspirin, acetaminophen, or nonsteroidal anti-inflammatory drugs (NSAIDs) are enough to suppress it. A cup of regular coffee is also frequently helpful.

If the headache is very severe and lasts for an unacceptably long time, many patients will go to the emergency room for relief. There they will usually receive an intravenous or intramuscular narcotic to take the pain away (they cannot take a pill because of the vomiting), together with dihydroergotamine, which has to be given intravenously. Dihydroergotamine is a derivative of ergotamine, an old medication used for migraine, and since it produces constriction of the blood vessels, people with complicated migraine are generally not allowed to take it.

If a patient's headaches are severe but occur less than once a week, doctors will usually give the patient a prescription for a narcotic analgesic to be taken by mouth at home. This gives the patient control over her headaches and is less disruptive to her life than having to go to the emergency room frequently. Patients need to know that they may become addicted to narcotics, and they must not take such drugs more than once every three days.

Frequent use of narcotics and other painkillers may lead to the development of analgesic-dependent, or rebound, headaches. Many of the medications that are effective in controlling an occasional attack of migraine—like Fiorinal®, Fioricet®, and Excedrin®—contain relatively strong painkillers, sometimes combined with a barbiturate. If these drugs are taken daily, the body becomes dependent on or addicted to them.

The same can be said for the NSAIDs, like ibuprofen and naproxen (Aleve®). About four hours after the patient has taken the medication, the blood level of the analgesic drops and the headache returns because the dependency "wants" the patient to take more medication. Anyone taking prescription or over-the-counter migraine pills three times daily for months has analgesic-dependent headaches. The only way to cure these is to wean patient off the medication gradually, while using medications like valproate or topiramate to prevent migraine attacks from coming.

Serotonin, a chemical present in the brain and in blood platelets, plays an important role in migraine. Drugs in the triptan class, like sumatriptan (Imitrex®), rizatriptan (Maxalt®), and eletriptan (Relpax®), selectively stimulate serotonin receptors in the brain and cerebral blood vessels, thus helping suppress individual migraine headaches. Though these drugs may produce some side effects, such as a feeling of pressure in the chest, they are safer and more effective than ergotamine. They work best if taken as early as possible, either at the time of the visual aura for someone with classical migraine, or at the first sign of the headache in the case of common migraine. I like to combine one of these triptan medications with aspirin or naproxen (Aleve®).

## Tension Headaches

Just about everyone gets a tension headache from time to time. Working long hours under pressure, missing meals, and arguing with people tend to produce a headache centered over the brows and back of the head. Tension headaches may even be a form of migraine. They usually respond to rest, relaxation, and mild analgesics. The sufferer may experience a tight, bandlike pain around her head all day and every day. For some reason, this type of headache is more common in middle-aged women. Neurologists find that these patients are usually depressed. Their headaches usually respond to relaxation treatment and antidepressant medications.

Many TV advertisements show the muscles around the head and neck to be the origin of muscle tension headaches. These commercials may have been what led neurologists to think of using botulinum toxin (Botox®) injections to weaken these muscles. The injections turned out to be relatively effective for both migraine and tension headaches. Perhaps muscle tension is a significant part of the process producing the pain of migraine.

## Brain Tumors and Headaches

Some people who develop severe headaches, particularly if they do not normally have headaches, become concerned about the possibility of a brain tumor or aneurysm. These two conditions are extremely rare causes of headaches, however. People with brain tumors usually don't go to doctors complaining of headaches. Much more commonly they see the doctor because of epileptic seizures or trouble with speech, balance, or vision. However, tumors in deep parts of the brain that are not as "eloquent," such as the basal ganglia or hypothalamus, may signal their presence with headaches before other neurological problems develop.

A slow-growing tumor will eventually increase the pressure inside the skull (intracranial pressure) and give rise to headaches.

Hydrocephalus (water on the brain) and blood clots, such as a chronic subdural hematoma (a clot between the outer and inner coverings of the brain, resulting from a blow to the head), may also cause gradually worsening headaches.

The headache of raised intracranial pressure gradually develops and worsens over weeks or months. It is often worse in the morning, and as the condition progresses the headache may awaken the patient from sleep. The reason for this morning headache is that retention of fluid and carbon dioxide during sleep increases the intracranial pressure, so that at night the pressure rises above the critical level needed to produce a headache. Pain comes from stretching the meninges—the pain receptors in the coverings of the brain and in the main arteries entering the brain.

As the pressure inside the skull rises, it is transmitted to the optic nerves at the backs of the eyes. This pressure produces a swollen optic disc—a symptom called papilledema—that can be seen by a neurologist looking into the eyes with an ophthalmoscope. If the pressure in the optic disc becomes too high, the blood supply of the retina may be cut off, particularly when the patient stoops or gets up suddenly. These maneuvers cause a drop in blood pressure so that temporarily blood does not reach the retina, and the patient becomes blind for a few seconds to a minute. These are called transient obscurations of vision, and they are very important warning signs of critically raised intracranial pressure.

## Cerebral Aneurysms and Headaches

As I describe in Chapter 3, a cerebral aneurysm is a blowout on an artery within the skull. These aneurysms usually cause no symptoms unless they rupture, and many such aneurysm never burst. However, if one does rupture, then a potentially fatal subarachnoid hemorrhage results. Nevertheless, the most important thing that I always tell patients with headaches is that aneurysms *never* the cause of the sort of headache that they are complaining about.

# Headaches Due to Pain in Adjacent Structures

Infection of the nasal sinuses, called sinusitis, or infections of the teeth and middle ear, as well as glaucoma of the eye, may all cause headaches. The type of headache is very different in each of these conditions, and the diagnosis is usually obvious. As I mentioned before, what patients often call sinus headaches because they are over the brows are actually caused by migraine. Sometimes these patients will say, "Ah, but my headaches are truly due to my allergies and sinuses because they are always associated with congestion of my nose." I try to tell them that migraine causes congestion of the nasal mucosa, but they may not believe me until I show them that nasal decongestant medicines don't help, while migraine medications prevent the headaches.

Any form of arthritis of the neck, such as rheumatoid arthritis or the wear-and-tear condition called cervical spondylosis, may cause headaches that usually start at the back of the head. The usual treatment is to wear a cervical (neck) collar for a month to decrease neck movements and to let the inflamed joints heal. A nerve at the back of the head, the occipital nerve, can be pinched as it goes through the occipital muscle. This causes a condition called occipital neuralgia, which can be treated by injections of steroids around the nerve.

Meningitis, an infectious inflammation of the meninges covering the brain, is a very serious cause of acute headaches and, like subarachnoid hemorrhage, needs immediate medical attention. Meningitis may be caused by a virus, in which case it will get better on its own, though the patient will need a spinal tap to be sure of the diagnosis. On the other hand, bacterial causes of meningitis are potentially lethal and need intensive treatment with the appropriate antibiotic to which the bug is sensitive. Meningococcal meningitis can occur in small epidemics in schools and camps, and it may be very rapidly fatal unless the diagnosis is made quickly; luckily, this bug is very sensitive to antibiotics. Tuberculous meningitis (that is, meningitis due to TB) is much slower to develop but can be equally fatal.

# Headache Due to Inflammation of the Arteries

New-onset headaches in anyone over the age of sixty need to be investigated with some degree of urgency by a doctor. Some of these patients turn out to have a brain tumor or other space-occupying lesions causing increase in the pressure inside the skull. Others may just have late-onset migraine, tension headaches, or headaches coming from arthritis in the neck. It is therefore crucial to get to the correct diagnosis.

One dangerous condition is temporal or cranial arteritis. This inflammatory disease of the arteries particularly affects people in the head. The headache usually localizes to the temples, and the doctor may find that the temporal arteries are thickened and tender. If a small piece of one of these thickened arteries is removed in a surgical biopsy, the pathologist will find inflammation. Besides the headache, the patient often has a generalized feeling of being unwell and uninterested in food, and he may complain of diffuse aching of the muscles. Blood tests that reveal the presence of an inflammatory process will be positive, thus adding to certainty about the diagnosis.

The main risk of leaving this arteritis undiagnosed and untreated is that the inflammation may lead to clotting and block the central retinal artery (the small artery going to the eye), causing sudden and permanent blindness in that eye. The arteries supplying the brain also can become blocked as a result of the inflammation, and a stroke might ensue.

A doctor who diagnoses cranial arteritis will usually treat the patient with high-dose steroids, usually prednisone, and will do so even before the blood test results have come back. It would be terrible if the patient went blind while waiting for the results! The arterial inflammation is usually rapidly responsive to prednisone, and the headaches disappear within a day or two. The steroid treatment must be continued until the inflammation burns itself out. The doctor will gradually reduce the dose while watching to see if the headaches return or if the blood tests for inflammation become abnormal again. If the steroid can be stopped without either of these things happening, then the patient is cured. This may take six months or more of treatment.

# Trigeminal Neuralgia

People with trigeminal neuralgia have attacks in which they suffer recurrent shoots of pain that cause them to cry out because it is so severe. They describe the pain as being like someone sticking a knife or a red-hot needle into their face. The pains are usually restricted to one side and may affect the upper, middle, and lower part of the face. The pain is so sharp that the patient winces, hence the name *tic douloureux* (which translates as "painful twitch"). The pain is usually brief, lasting only one or two seconds, but it recurs many times a day. It can be precipitated by touching the face or the inside of the mouth. Even a soft breath on the cheek can cause a flash of pain. The place where a stimulus may cause a shoot of pain is called a trigger zone.

Trigeminal neuralgia comes in attacks that last for weeks or months and then disappear for months or even years, though they usually recur. While they are in an attack, patients will not eat, shave, or touch their faces—whatever is their particular trigger.

The pain of trigeminal neuralgia happens when something irritates the trigeminal nerve root where it enters the brain stem near the base of the skull. Whatever causes the irritation, it induces a spontaneous discharge of impulses that shoot up to the pain centers of the brain. This is called a generator potential, and it develops in an area of demyelination in the trigeminal sensory nerve fibers—spots where the nerve fibers are naked because of damage to their myelin sheaths.

The typical patient with trigeminal neuralgia is a man or woman in his or her senior years without any easily demonstrated cause for the painful condition, such as a meningioma pressing on the trigeminal nerve. In the elderly a small artery beating against the trigeminal nerve root is often thought to be responsible for producing irritation of the trigeminal nerve. A neurosurgical procedure to put a cushion between the artery and the nerve is often curative for the typical elderly patient with this condition, but this is major surgery. A younger patient with trigeminal neuralgia, particularly a woman, usually has multiple sclerosis, and a plaque of demyelination just where the trigeminal nerve enters the brain stem is irritating the nerve.

Antiepileptic drugs like carbamazepine (Tegretol®) are quite effective in suppressing trigeminal attacks, and thus most people can avoid surgery. The older neurosurgical procedure of cutting the trigeminal nerve root is still required in some cases. Injection of alcohol or glycerine into the trigeminal ganglion, as well as focused irradiation using the Gamma Knife® or CyberKnife®, are other ways of preventing the episodes of pain that characterize trigeminal neuralgia.

# Low-pressure Headaches

Since the invention of the spinal tap (lumbar puncture, or LP) by Heinrich Quincke in 1891, we have found that up to 10 percent of patients get a characteristic headache, called a post-LP headache, in the wake of the procedure. This is one of the reasons that patients shy away from having LPs if they can. Post-LP headache is caused by low pressure of the CSF that results from a small hole in the fibrous sac at the bottom of the spine, called the dural sac, through which CSF leaks following a spinal tap. The low-pressure headache characteristically develops when the patient sits or stands, and patients find relief by lying down. The low pressure allows the brain to sag toward the base of the skull whenever the patient sits up, thus stretching the pain-producing structures within the skull.

There are several ways to reduce the risk of a post-LP headache. A thin needle that does not cut the fibers of the dura undoubtedly helps. If the doctor is skillful and needs only a single attempt to get the sample of CSF, he will leave only one hole in the dura, while if he is less skillful he may leave multiple holes to leak. After an LP, the patient should rest in bed on his belly for an hour; lying on the belly helps seal off the hole in the dura. The patient should take lots of fluid and caffeine, which seem to stimulate the production of CSF.

Despite all these precautions, if the patient gets a headache when he stands, he should lay down for a further twenty-four hours and repeat the other parts of the prevention plan. Medications to kill the pain are also important. Occasionally, if the headache continues for days, then a "magic bullet" called a blood patch is needed. Some of the patient's own blood is drawn from a vein and injected into the space outside the dural sac at the site of the original lumbar puncture. The blood compresses the hole in the dura and prevents further leakage of CSF.

Occasionally, low-pressure headaches develop spontaneously, without a spinal tap. This happens when a spontaneous rupture of a small cyst on a nerve root allows CSF to leak out. Surgical closure of this dural fistula is needed if it does not seal spontaneously.

## High-altitude Headaches

Dentists are well aware that if patients with a tooth root infection, called an apical abscess, go up in an aircraft they may develop severe dental pain. Inside the abscess is a small bubble of gas, which expands as the cabin pressure is lowered at altitude. A blocked nasal sinus may cause similar pain. It also may happen if a person cannot clear her ears because the Eustachian tube going to the middle ear is blocked.

About 20 percent of people get bad migraine-type headaches at high altitudes (over 12,000 feet), perhaps because the small amount of oxygen in the air makes the arteries of the brain dilate to get more oxygen to where it is needed. People sleeping in ski lodges at an altitude above 9,000 feet frequently wake up with headaches. Acetazolamide (Diamox®) helps prevent these headaches. This drug blocks an enzyme called carbonic anhydrase, which plays an important role in the secretion of CSF; it therefore lowers the pressure of the CSF inside the head. The only problem is that acetazolamide produces a pins-and-needles sensation in the hands, feet, and face in about 20 percent of people.

I had two patients who suffered terrible head pains every time they went up in an aircraft. The first was an attorney, who had traveled in aircraft for many years without problems. A year before he came to see me, he started getting excruciating pain in the eye and forehead on one side whenever the plane reached 20,000 feet. The pains became so bad that he gave up flying and was unable to take up a seat on the board of the American Bar Association as a result.

The other patient was the wife of a successful businessman. She used to enjoy traveling with her husband and had flown commercially for many years. For no reason, she started getting bilateral severe pain across her forehead at about 20,000 feet. Both patients said that the first time they developed the pain it was so bad that they had been reduced to tears and had screamed for the flight attendant. The pilot had brought the plane down to a lower altitude, and this relieved the pain.

Neither patient had any nervous system abnormalities, and their MRIs were absolutely normal. Neither patient had any dental or ear, nose, or throat cause of the pain. I wanted to research the relationship between altitude and the pain since commercial airline cabins are depressurized to an altitude of only about 8,000 feet (that is, to the pressure that would be experienced at 8,000 feet about sea level), which seems relatively low to produce such a decompression syndrome. However, I couldn't persuade officials in the space medicine facilities of the U.S. Air Force to allow me to bring in the patients for study.

These head pains threatened to ruin the lives of both of my patients. The lawyer eventually underwent a surgical procedure to cut the nerve that carries pain messages from the sinuses around his nose to the brain on the side of the pain. This cured his condition for several years, though the altitude-related pain returned—presumably because the nerve grew back—and surgery was again needed to cure the pain.

The other patient has found that a pain-blocking antiepileptic medication, gabapentin (Neurontin®), prevents the pain if she takes a large enough dose an hour before the flight and repeats it every four hours during long flights. Both of my patients are very happy to be free of the altitude headaches. Like many of my chronic migraine sufferers who have benefited from effective treatment for their headaches, they told me that they felt that they had been given back control of their lives.

## Chapter 12

# Peripheral Neuropathies and Carpal Tunnel Syndrome

Terry was a forty-one-year-old man who was admitted to my hospital neurology service because of severe leg weakness that had been worsening for four months. He was now almost unable to walk. He only sought medical attention when he could not walk because he had no health insurance.

My residents thought that Terry had a condition called Charcot-Marie-Tooth (CMT) disease because he had severe weakness of the muscles below the knees and a marked foot drop. When I questioned Terry, I found that he knew of no one else in his family with a similar condition. This made me suspicious of the diagnosis, since CMT is usually inherited. When I examined Terry, I found that there was very little wasting of the muscles below the knees, despite the severe weakness that affected not just the muscles that move the ankles but also the muscles that flex the hips.

I told the residents that this pattern of weakness without much muscle atrophy suggested that the diagnosis was not CMT but rather chronic inflammatory demyelinating polyneuropathy (CIDP). I emphasized that, as is not the case with CMT, we can treat CIDP. I felt rather proud of myself when nerve conduction studies and a nerve biopsy confirmed the diagnosis of CIDP—but, as we all know, pride comes before a fall.

CIDP is an autoimmune disease in which the body produces antibodies against its own nerves. We therefore treated Terry with a steroid, prednisone. At first he got remarkably better and walked out of the hospital. However, over the next three years steroids began to lose their effect, and Terry required additional treatment (which I will discuss later) to keep the disease under control. Eventually, we were unable to control the neuropathy and the disease spread to his arms. He became bedridden and unable to feed himself.

We readmitted Terry to the hospital, and when a new set of residents went through the hospital records from his previous admission, they discovered that one of the test results, a report of the blood immuno-electrophoresis study (investigation of the proteins in the blood), had not come back while Terry was in the hospital that first time. It had been filed in the chart and not seen by the people looking after him. The abnormal immunoelectrophoresis test suggested that Terry had a myeloma, a type of bone marrow cancer, which in turn had caused the CIDP.

We X-rayed Terry's bones, found several lesions suggesting multiple myeloma, and confirming the diagnosis with a biopsy. We gave him radiation and chemotherapy, and after two months he began to improve. We continued the chemotherapy for six months, and a year later, the only problem that remained was weakness of the muscles below his knees, for which he needed a brace.

Terry's case taught me several lessons. We must always search for an underlying cause of neuropathy in CIDP, and we must insist on seeing every test result before deciding that a neuropathy has no cause.

## What Is Peripheral Neuropathy?

As I describe in Chapter 1, the peripheral nervous system is made up of all the nerves outside the brain and spinal cord. It carries signals back and forth between the brain and the rest of the body. The peripheral nerves are longer, more numerous, and less protected than those of the brain and spinal cord. They are subject to many different diseases that are grouped under the term *peripheral neuropathy* (*neuropathy* refers to any disease or injury of the peripheral nerves).

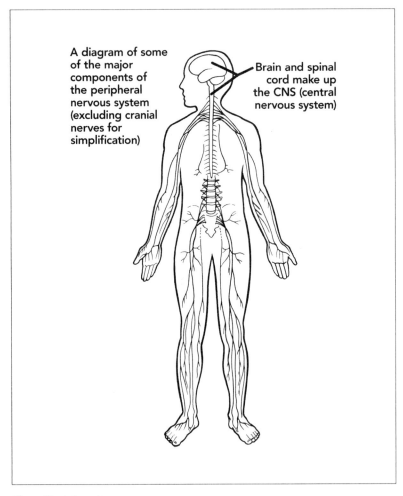

A diagram of some of the major components of the peripheral nervous system (excluding cranial nerves for simplification)

Brain and spinal cord make up the CNS (central nervous system)

*Fig. 9:* **Peripheral nervous system**

Peripheral neuropathies are diseases of the peripheral nerves, which comprise all of the nervous system except for the brain and spinal cord.

Diagnosing of the commonest causes of peripheral neuropathy, such as diabetic neuropathy or a pinched nerve, is relatively easy. For the less common causes of peripheral neuropathy, of which there are thousands, finding the diagnosis is like searching for a needle in a haystack. When faced with this task, many neurologists throw up their hands and refer the patient to one of the small number of neurologists who specialize in peripheral neuropathies.

The Neuropathy Association estimates that there are 20 million cases of peripheral neuropathy in the United States, and this may well be an underestimate. A significant neuropathy occurs as a complication in up to 5 percent of people with diabetes, meaning that there are over a million patients with diabetic neuropathy in the United States. Hereditary neuropathies occur in about one in twenty-five hundred of the general population. Carpal tunnel syndrome (CTS) occurs in one in twenty of the population and, among people who are at high risk—such as people with arthritis or people who work their wrists repetitively, the rate of occurrence is ten times greater. Leprosy is the commonest cause of peripheral neuropathy worldwide; a quarter of a billion new cases are diagnosed each year, most of them in India and Brazil.

Nerves are delicate and easily damaged. For instance, the sciatic nerve, which starts in the lower back and goes all the way down to the toes, can be damaged by a bullet wound or caught between the broken ends of a fractured femur. The resulting paralysis of the foot and loss of sensation below the knee is termed a sciatic neuropathy. This is one example of a mononeuropathy, a neuropathy in which only one nerve is damaged.

The nerves are often injured because of where they lie in the body. This is particularly true of the nerves in the arm because we use our arms in all sorts of risky activities. The ulnar nerve, which runs down the inside of the arm behind the elbow and into the hand, is easily damaged where it lies in a bony groove at the back of the elbow. When it is hit, it sends an unpleasant tingling pain to the brain; this is what we call hitting your funny bone.

Similarly, the median nerve that runs down the front of the arm to the hand is easily compressed as it goes through the carpal tunnel at the front of the wrist. This is the usual cause of waking in the night with painful tingling in the hand that feels as though it has "gone to sleep." CTS is the most common cause of a pinched nerve, also called a nerve compression or entrapment neuropathy. A pinched nerve is painful, as anyone who has a herniated disc pressing on a nerve root can testify.

Neurologists classify peripheral neuropathies according to the type of nerve fiber that is involved. In most patients with damage to the peripheral nerves, the motor, sensory, and autonomic nerve fibers are all involved. We call this a mixed sensory-motor neuropathy. If the motor nerve fibers are preferentially damaged, we call it a motor neuropathy. Some forms of CMT disease are predominantly motor neuropathies. In rare cases the autonomic nerve fibers are particularly damaged, producing an autonomic neuropathy, such as a familial amyloid neuropathy, which I will describe later.

Diseases that affect only the sensory nerve fibers are called sensory neuropathies. Different types of sensation can be lost depending upon what specific type or diameter of sensory fiber is involved. For example, a large fiber sensory neuropathy causes loss of the person's ability to feel a vibration, a light touch, or the position of a joint; the patient will often feel pins and needles (paresthesias) and jolts of lightning-like pain. Diseases that affect unmyelinated sensory fiber cause loss of the ability to detect pain and temperature. These small fiber sensory neuropathies often result in the fibers spontaneously discharging and sending nerve impulses to the brain, which interprets them as a burning sensation in the body part supplied by these unmyelinated fibers.

Some peripheral neuropathies come on rapidly or, at the most, within a few weeks. They are called acute polyneuropathies. Guillain-Barré syndrome is such a disease. Much more common are chronic polyneuropathies that develop over months, years, or even decades, such as CMT disease and CIDP, which my patient Terry suffered from.

In my book for neurologists, *Neurology in Clinical Practice*, peripheral nerves and their diseases take up 107 pages, but I think that my description here and in Chapter 1 should enable you to understand why peripheral neuropathies are so complex. There may be a thousand different causes of peripheral neuropathy, and we know only five hundred of them. The remainder of cases are described as idiopathic— that is, without a known cause.

## Tests for Diagnosing Peripheral Nerve Disease

Peripheral neuropathies are relatively easy to recognize, but it is a daunting task to determine their cause. Neurologists who are good at diagnosing the cause of peripheral neuropathies know that different diseases produce different patterns of nerve damage, and therefore the pattern helps them identify the culprit. They also make wise use of laboratory tests. I use the word "wise" *because* the neurologist must understand each test and know what tests are needed for each pattern of disease. It is not sensible or cost-effective to put patients through a hundred different tests, most of which have no hope of revealing the cause.

The first investigation of a patient with a peripheral nerve problem is the interview and examination by a neurologist experienced in peripheral neuromuscular diseases. This reveals the nerves and muscles involved and the type of nerve fibers that are damaged. At the end of the examination the neuromuscular specialist should have a good idea as to what type of nerve disease is likely to be the cause of the condition, as well as what further investigations will be needed to discover the cause.

Many medications and recreational drugs can damage the nerves and produce toxic neuropathies. An astute neurologist will question the patient about what medications he was taking when he developed the symptoms of neuropathy. He will also ask about recreational drugs, with the knowledge that it is often difficult to get a straight answer. Alcohol is the commonest "social neurotoxin," and often patients need to be quizzed very intensely before they reveal the exact amount of alcohol they consume.

An example of the type of detective work needed to reveal a history of recreational drug use is the case of a dentist in his early forties, who came to see me complaining of numbness of the feet and hands and great difficulty walking. He had signs of a peripheral polyneuropathy affecting the large-diameter myelinated fibers—that is, he had weakness and wasting of the muscles moving his feet and fingers, and he could not feel light touch, vibration, or small movements of the joints in his hands and feet. In addition, he had spasticity and abnormally brisk tendon reflexes, which indicated spinal cord damage. These signs suggested that vitamin $B_{12}$ deficiency was a likely cause of his condition. However, his vitamin $B_{12}$ level and tests for malabsorption of vitamin $B_{12}$ were negative, and he did not improve with vitamin $B_{12}$ injections.

When the dentist came back to see me, I realized that he seemed less bright than a dentist should be. With my suspicions aroused, I took his girlfriend aside to ask if she could tell me what might be causing his condition. She broke down in tears and told me the whole story. Every weekend for the last two years he would strap himself to his dental chair, put a mask over his face, and inhale nitrous oxide (also called laughing gas). She said that originally he only did this for a few hours a day, but gradually he had increased the duration to most of the weekend. Lately he had complained he was not getting the same high, so he had cut the oxygen concentration in the gas from the normal 20 percent to 10 percent.

My patient was suffering damage to both his nerves and his brain due to abuse of nitrous oxide that blocked vitamin $B_{12}$ and lack of oxygen. I confronted him, pointing out that he was going to become paralyzed and demented if he went on abusing nitrous oxide, and eventually he stopped. His neurological condition improved slowly but he still needed a cane to walk. A few months later a medical journal article reported several similar cases, and we now know that nitrous oxide blocks enzymes involved in vitamin $B_{12}$ metabolism.

## Blood tests

The commonest cause of a polyneuropathy in developed countries is diabetes mellitus. Doctors diagnose diabetes via a blood test for either fasting blood sugar level or hemoglobin A1c level (an index of a person's blood sugar level over the past few weeks). If either level is abnormally high, the doctor will do a glucose tolerance test, in which he has the patient drink 50 grams of glucose and draws blood for glucose levels every half hour for three hours. Many patients will find that they have borderline diabetes. The crucial question is whether diabetes is relevant as the cause of their neuropathy or just a chance finding that might be present in someone else without causing any problem with the peripheral nerves.

The neurologist trying to find the cause of a neuropathy will arrange a standard series of hematological and biochemical screening blood tests. These will detect evidence of many of the medical diseases that may damage the peripheral nerves, including chronic kidney and liver failure, inflammation of the arteries going to the nerves (vasculitis), vitamin $B_{12}$ deficiency, low thyroid activity (hypothyroidism), leukemia, and a bone marrow cancer such as myeloma.

One of the tests for myeloma is the plasma immunoelectrophoresis study that we missed upon Terry's first admission to the hospital. This may show an abnormal protein that is classified as a gamma globulin, and thus the patient is said to have a gammopathy. The most sensitive test for gammopathy is a refinement of immunoelectrophoresis called immunofixation. In some patients with Terry's condition, CIDP, this test is positive, and the neuropathy will usually respond to treatment, as I indicated earlier.

Some peripheral nerve diseases are inherited; CMT disease is the commonest. If the patient knows that other members of his family had a condition similar to his, then the neurologist may arrange DNA tests. Several commercial laboratories offer these gene tests for a comprehensive charge of several thousand dollars. Though a positive test eliminates the need for further tests and is important for genetic counseling, it must be remembered that none of the forms of CMT disease is yet treatable.

If the patient has no family history and if the screening blood tests did not reveal the underlying cause of the neuropathy, a more focused approach is needed. This is where a general neurologist may become lost and seek help from laboratories that offer diagnostic neuropathy screening tests. These tests are very expensive, usually negative, and rarely needed, since the clinical clues should have told the doctor that the diseases that they test for are very unlikely to be the cause of the neuropathy in this particular patient. The tests are often done "because we can," without thought to the likelihood of a positive result or to the cost.

## Nerve conduction studies and electromyography

Knowing the conduction speed of nerve fibers can be of help in determining the type of damage in a peripheral polyneuropathy. Medical personnel test nerve conduction by stimulating the nerves with tiny, but still slightly painful, electric shocks to make the muscle supplied by that nerve twitch. If the nerve is stimulated at one point at a place at a distance from a muscle—say, the elbow—and at another point close to the muscle—say, the wrist—and if the time that it takes for the impulse to get from the first to the second stimulus point is measured on a monitor, then it is possible to calculate the speed of nerve conduction. This is called a nerve conduction velocity (NCV) test.

The spike that will be recorded on the computer monitor is called the evoked muscle action potential. It is a measure of the number of motor nerve fibers going to the muscle. Loss of motor nerve fibers will decrease the height of the "spike"—the muscle action potential amplitude.

If there is loss of myelin sheaths from the nerve fibers, nerve conduction velocity will decrease from the normal maximum of forty-five to fifty meters per second to below about thirty-five meters per second. Disease of the axons generally does not affect the maximum conduction speed, while a severe demyelinating neuropathy may reduce the conduction velocity to as low as five meters per second. As we have seen, demyelination may be seen in both inherited and inflammatory nerve diseases.

The electromyogram (EMG) is used to reveal loss of motor nerve fibers going to muscles, a process called denervation. The doctor looks for electrical changes in the muscle by inserting a thin recording needle electrode into the main bulk of the muscle. The electrical potentials produced by the muscle fibers are shown on a monitor and played over a loudspeaker. When the person is at rest, no electrical activity should be coming from the muscle fibers, but if there is denervation then the potentials produce a sound like fat frying in the pan, and the screen shows short, low voltage potentials called fibrillation potentials. When the patient contracts his muscle slightly, the monitor screen begins to show individual motor units (a motor unit is defined as one motor neuron plus all the muscle fibers that it innervates). The shape of these motor units is different in denervated muscle when compared with normal muscle. Motor unit potentials in partly denervated muscle are typically larger in height (amplitude) and width (duration). On the other hand, motor unit potentials in a patient with a muscle disease like muscular dystrophy are abnormally small, both in height and in width.

An expert neurologist will use the NCV and EMG tests like a detective to probe the exact place and type of nerve injury. For instance, if these tests show damage to the nerve fibers of the L3 lumbar nerve root, the neurologist will be able to tell the neurosurgeon not to operate on the L5-S1 disc that an MRI scan might have shown to be herniated. Similarly, in a patient with arm pain, the NCV and EMG tests may reveal that the patient's problems come from damage in the nerves at the junction of the arm and the shoulder, rather than in the disc in the neck seen on the CT scan. The NCV and EMG tests can separate a disease of the muscles, like muscular dystrophy, from a disease of the motor neurons, like ALS.

These electrical tests are also useful in following the condition's course and indicating the prognosis. For example, a facial nerve paralysis, also called Bell's palsy, may show no evidence of recovery after three weeks, thus leading the doctor to think that the prognosis is bleak. In some cases, this is correct because the axons in the nerve have all degenerated. However, in other cases, if the NCV study shows that the facial nerve axons can still be stimulated, the paralysis is the result of demyelination, which stops nerve impulses from proceeding down the nerve, and the prognosis is much better.

## X-ray and imaging studies

A hidden cancer somewhere in the body may cause several types of neuropathy, called paraneoplastic neuropathies. Thus, screening with X-rays and CT or MRI scans of the chest, abdomen, and pelvis is sometimes needed.

## Nerve biopsy

The commonest cause of peripheral polyneuropathy is leprosy. A neurologist suspecting leprosy will order a nerve biopsy and skin scrapings. These may reveal the presence of the bacterium that causes leprosy. The nerve biopsy may show the changes in structure that are typical of leprosy, as well as the presence of leprosy bacilli. However, in regions of the world where leprosy is common, doctors can make this diagnosis simply by seeing the typical picture of a neuropathy.

Many doctors think that a nerve biopsy is needed in order to come to the final diagnosis of a peripheral neuropathy. This is not true; in most cases, a biopsy will not show us the exact cause of the neuropathy. The conditions that may be diagnosed via nerve biopsy are vasculitis, leprosy, a few of the autoimmune polyneuropathies, and a few of the hereditary neuropathies.

If a doctor considers one of the conditions that can be identified on a nerve biopsy, he usually asks a surgeon to biopsy the sural nerve, which lies at the back of the ankle bone called the lateral malleolus. This nerve is used because it is a sensory nerve, and its removal produces only a small numb patch on the outside of the foot. However, an occasional patient will be left with a painful scar or chronic pain in the foot.

If a neurologist recommends a nerve biopsy, it is generally best for the patient to go to a specialized neuromuscular neurologist. This specialist will be better able to decide if a nerve biopsy is needed, and he will also have access to a pathology laboratory that uses all the modern techniques needed to study nerve biopsies. Moreover, the surgeons doing nerve biopsies in these specialized centers are experienced in taking just a thin sliver (called a fascicular biopsy) of the sural nerve. They are even able to take a fascicular biopsy of a mixed nerve (like the common peroneal nerve at the outer side of the knee) without producing muscle weakness.

# Causes of Peripheral Nerve Disease

The symptoms of peripheral nerve disease are easy to understand. If the sensory nerve fibers are damaged, there will be loss of sensation. In addition, a person with sensory fiber damage may feel pain because of spontaneous discharges of nerve impulses from the site of damage, which the brain interprets as pain. The type of pain and the details of the sensory loss depend on which type of sensory nerve fiber is involved. If the motor nerve fibers are involved, there will be weakness and wasting of muscles. There may also be spontaneous twitching of muscles, called fasciculations, as a result of spontaneous discharges of the sick motor nerve cells.

*Acute neuropathies*

Hyperacute mononeuropathies (damage to one nerve) result from direct trauma to a nerve or from inflammation of a blood vessel going to that nerve (a vasculitis). The inflammation causes the blood in the artery to clot, producing blockage of the artery. The result is a "nerve stroke." Typically a vasculitis will produce a nerve stroke affecting several single nerves, one after the other; the term *multiple mononeuropathy* is given to this pattern of peripheral nerve disease. For example, the patient may get a foot drop from damage to the peroneal nerve at the knee, followed two or three weeks later by a wrist drop due to radial nerve damage. Diabetes can produce a similar picture to a vasculitis because it damages the small blood vessels in the nerves.

## Guillain-Barré syndrome (GBS)

Guillain-Barré syndrome is sometimes termed an acute polyneuropathy, because the neurological problem develops over a few days or, at maximum, four weeks. Another name is acute inflammatory demyelinating polyneuropathy (AIDP). Typically, the patient develops tingling in his feet and heaviness in his legs. These symptoms gradually worsen and spread upward, leading to paralysis of much of the body in a few days to four weeks. In about 10 percent of patients the polyneuropathy progresses to complete paralysis, with quadriplegia and respiratory failure requiring ventilator support.

It must be terrifying for a previously healthy person to be struck down suddenly by GBS. The only good part about it is that more than 90 percent of people eventually make a complete recovery, though this may take up to two years if the paralysis was severe. I always tell GBS patients about the good prognosis when they come into the hospital and are terrified that they will remain paralyzed for life. This led to one of my most embarrassing moments as a neurologist.

Soon after I came to the United States, I was teaching residents at the bedside of a young man with GBS. After completing the teaching, I gave him my standard reassurance about the good prognosis and left him with the encouraging words that are used in Britain in this situation: "Keep your pecker up." It took some time for the residents and nurses to stop laughing and to explain to me the American use of the word *pecker*, which is quite different from its use in England to describe the nose.

GBS is an autoimmune disease in which the body produces antibodies that damage the myelin of the peripheral nerves. When the myelin breaks down, it causes what is called a demyelinating neuropathy. In the pure condition, demyelination leaves the axon intact. Since the Schwann cells form myelin and reestablish nerve conduction quite quickly after the antibodies have disappeared, some patients with GBS recover within a few weeks. However, in other patients, the antibodies call in inflammatory cells to help them attack the myelin, and the axons also get damaged. In this case, the patient with GBS remains paralyzed much longer because the axons are regenerating at only one millimeter per day.

Many patients who develop GBS had a gastrointestinal infection or immunization a few weeks earlier. The immune system probably produces antibodies to these stimuli that cross-react with peripheral nerve myelin to cause demyelination. Recovery begins when the antibodies and secondary inflammatory cells in the nerves disappear and new myelin starts to be formed.

In 1916 French neurologists Georges Guillain, Jean-Alexandre Barré, and André Strohl first clearly characterized this disease in French soldiers during World War I, and thereafter it became known by the name of the first two authors. The spinal tap and the accompanying examination of the CSF, were just coming into use at that time, and the three doctors reported increased protein in the CSF without an increased white cell count in their patients. They were struck by the difference between what they saw in their syndrome and the CSF from patients with meningitis, where both protein and white cells are increased. This dissociation between the concentration of protein and white cells is still used as an aid to the diagnosis of GBS.

GBS is now treated with either plasmapheresis (also called plasma exchange) or high-dose intravenous immunoglobulin (IVIg). Plasma exchange is almost the opposite of infusing immunoglobulins, for it takes out substances from the blood, rather like kidney dialysis. The blood is taken out of one of the patient's veins; the red cells are spun off from the plasma in a centrifuge and then resuspended in saline; the plasma containing the harmful antibodies is discarded; and the red cells are then run back into another of the patient's veins. IVIg is produced by purifying the antibody fraction (called immunoglobulin) from hundreds of bottles of blood from donors. This thick, protein-rich liquid somehow blocks the antibodies that are causing GBS.

We now know that both of these treatments slightly speed up recovery from GBS, though the response is highly variable, as I learned when I was involved in the placebo-controlled trials of plasma exchange. One of our medical students came into the hospital having lost his ability to walk in a period of a few days due to GBS. We drew a card assigning him to one or the other of the two groups in the trial— placebo or active treatment. The next day, we were gratified to find that he was starting to walk again, and he made a remarkably rapid recovery. If he had drawn plasma exchange as his treatment group we would have ascribed the rapid response to the treatment, but in fact he drew the other card—"No plasma exchange."

## Diseases damaging the nerve plexuses

The nerve plexuses lie between the nerves of the limbs and the nerve roots as they run through the subarachnoid space within the spinal canal on their way to join the spinal cord. Conditions damaging the nerve plexuses are called plexopathies. The brachial plexus is in the root of the neck, and the lumbosacral plexus lies in the back wall of the abdominal cavity. In these plexuses, nerves branch, join, and rebranch in a seemingly random fashion (though in fact it is well organized). The function of nerve plexuses is to ensure that an injury of one part of the plexus will not completely destroy the nerve supply to any one muscle or area of skin. This function follows the principle of multiple redundancy. In an injury of one of the plexuses, some surviving nerve fibers running through undamaged parts will allow at least partial residual function.

The plexuses may be damaged by a bullet or stab wound, by fractures of bones in the area, by vasculitis, and by cancerous invasion. Radiation therapy of a local cancer may also damage the plexuses. Diabetes may cause a painful lumbosacral plexopathy.

In addition, either the brachial or the lumbosacral plexus may suffer damage without any known cause. This is very perplexing to doctors and usually very painful for the patient. It is likely that the damage is caused by an autoimmune inflammation, but why this attacks only the plexuses and not the rest of the peripheral nerves is unknown. The only treatment is to keep the pain under control until the inflammation abates and the plexopathy recovers spontaneously. Patients often suffer significant paralysis of the muscles of the arm or leg supplied by the damaged plexus, but this will generally recover in six to twenty-four months.

## Chronic polyneuropathies

Chronic polyneuropathies are responsible for 90 percent of peripheral nerve disease cases. Unfortunately for nearly half the affected patients, the cause of the polyneuropathy is not found. These patients are said to have idiopathic chronic polyneuropathy. The typical picture is a very slow development of motor and sensory loss starting in the feet, spreading up the legs, and later affecting the fingers and hands. The weakness and wasting of the leg muscles leads to a foot drop; the patient cannot lift his toes when climbing stairs and often cannot rise up on his toes. The patient will often trip on curbs and stairs as a result of this foot drop. With his eyes closed, the patient will often be unable to tell whether his finger is being moved up or down by the neurologist. Pin prick, temperature, light touch, and vibration sensation may all be reduced in the hands, feet, and legs. The tendon reflexes are often lost in a patient with peripheral polyneuropathy.

Several specific features of individual chronic polyneuropathies can help experienced neuromuscular neurologists come to a diagnosis. These are the "pearls" that senior neurologists like to teach their trainees. I will mention a few of these as we go through the diseases.

## Familial polyneuropathies

A few polyneuropathies run in families. These conditions may be dominantly or recessively inherited. In dominant conditions, one of the parents also had the disease, and half the siblings are likely to develop it. In recessive conditions, sometimes there has been inbreeding—for instance, marriage between first cousins—and, though neither parent is affected, one-quarter of the siblings is likely to have the same condition.

The commonest hereditary neuropathy is CMT disease, though it is in fact a whole group of conditions that produce a similar chronic polyneuropathy. The condition is also called peroneal muscular atrophy because of the wasting of the muscles at the front of the shins (the peroneal muscles). This group of familial diseases was first reported in two separate publications in 1886, one by Jean-Martin Charcot and Pierre Marie in France, and the other by an English physician Howard Tooth. Though the name Charcot-Marie-Tooth disease, or CMT, is now embedded in our medical language, it often confuses patients, several of whom have exclaimed, "But I don't have problems with my teeth!"

CMT is a very slowly progressive polyneuropathy. Because it affects motor fibers more than sensory ones, muscle wasting and weakness are the main problems. It is a length-dependent, dying-back condition, as I describe in Chapter 1, so that the weakness first starts in the small muscles of the feet, causing children to develop high arches and hammer toes. Cramps in the feet are frequent. In early adult life, symptoms of muscle weakness become more prominent, and the person begins to trip due to the development of a foot drop.

Over the next two or three decades, weakness spreads to the hands, and muscle wasting and distortion of the positions of the fingers results in a clawlike position. The neurologist may find that the patient has lost perception of a pin prick and light touch up to the knees and on the fingers. Occasionally, the patient's voice may be hoarse because of dying back of nerves that go to the vocal cords.

There are two main types of CMT disease. In axonal polyneuropathy, the axons of the nerves are damaged by the disease. In this type of condition, as I explained in the section on tests, the conduction speed of the remaining nerve fibers is normal at about 45 to 50 meters per second. In demyelinating polyneuropathy, the other type of CMT, the myelin is most affected. In patients with this type of CMT, nerve conduction studies reveal very slow velocities of five to twenty meters per second. The demyelinating forms make up about two-thirds of the patients with CMT disease, while the axonal forms comprise about one-third. Genetic mutations have been detected in 75 percent of patients with the demyelinating forms, but so far responsible genes have been identified in less than 20 percent of patients with axonal forms.

At present we have no specific medication to treat either of these inherited peripheral nerve diseases, though rehabilitation helps. This includes aids and appliances, like braces to prevent foot drop and canes, and walkers and wheelchairs to assist in mobility. There are also a few aids and appliances for impaired hand function. Genetic counseling plays an important role in helping a couple who might pass on a disease to their children to decide how to deal with this problem.

While CMT affects mainly the motor nerves, other familial diseases of peripheral nerves affect mainly the sensory fibers; these diseases are called hereditary sensory neuropathies. Because these patients lose sensation in their feet, they are liable to suffer injuries and infections without being aware of them. Patients often lose fingers, toes, and even a whole foot because of sensory loss. Leprosy can cause a similar problem.

Some inherited neuropathies are caused by enzyme deficiencies. Enzymes are specialized proteins, some of which break down compounds in cells. Deficiency of an enzyme may cause excess amounts of that compound to accumulate in the cells, and in the case of the peripheral nerves this can produce a polyneuropathy. Metachromatic leukodystrophy is caused by deficiency of the enzyme that breaks down excess sulfatide in the myelin sheaths. As a result, sulfatide accumulates and damages both the central and peripheral nervous systems. This neuropathy used to be diagnosed by a nerve biopsy, but now there is a blood test for confirming the diagnosis. Children experience a mixed sensory-motor polyneuropathy in the feet and hands, but soon they develop progressive spasticity and mental deterioration due to damage to the brain and spinal cord.

## Familial amyloid polyneuropathy

This condition is a dominantly inherited peripheral neuropathy caused by mutation of a gene for a protein that has absolutely nothing to do with peripheral nerves. The protein, transthyretin, is present in the blood and transports thyroid hormone and vitamin A to where they are needed. The mutation for familial amyloid polyneuropathy (Met30 mutation) causes the protein to change its structure and to form insoluble deposits that damage nerves and the sensory ganglia that lie on the nerve roots close to the spinal cord. This process of damaging the nerves is called a toxic gain of function by scientists investigating how a gene mutation causes disease; by this they mean that the mutant protein becomes toxic in a way totally unrelated to its normal function.

The mutant protein particularly damages the small sensory neurons and the autonomic neurons, so that patients lose pain and temperature sensation in the hands and feet, as well as autonomic functions, such as keeping the blood pressure high enough to prevent fainting when the patient is standing. Patients with this disease also lose control of the bowels and bladder, and men suffer loss of sexual function.

Transthyretin is made in the liver, and the only truly effective cure of familial amyloid polyneuropathy at present is liver transplantation, in which the patient's liver is replaced by a donor's liver that produces normal transthyretin. Liver transplantation has its own risks, and the transplantation has to be done early in the disease, because once enough mutant transthyretin has poisoned the nerves, the condition may be irreversible.

## Diabetic polyneuropathy

Of the more than twenty-five million people with diabetes in the United States, 5 percent have diabetic neuropathy, many without realizing it. Diabetes mellitus causes an increased blood sugar level due to decreased amount or action of insulin on the tissues. Type I diabetes is an autoimmune disease in which, for an unknown reason, the body produces autoantibodies that damage the insulin-producing pancreatic islet cells. Type II diabetes, by contrast, is a metabolic disorder in which the islet cells gradually lose the ability to make normal amounts of insulin, and the peripheral tissues also become resistant to the effects of the insulin. Recent research suggests that hormones secreted by the small intestine may play a role in Type II diabetes by altering the secretion of insulin and another hormone, glucagons, from the pancreas, as well as lowering the sensitivity of insulin receptors on cells like the peripheral nerves.

In both types of diabetes mellitus, the action of insulin on the peripheral nerves is reduced so that not enough glucose enters the axons and the Schwann cells of the nerve fibers. Nerve fiber nutrition is therefore impaired, and chronic nerve damage results. The symptoms of diabetic polyneuropathy usually begin with numbness and tingling in the toes that gradually spread up the legs. Nerve damage frequently affects the unmyelinated fibers more than the large myelinated nerve fibers. This causes the patient to lose pain and temperature sensation and to have distressing sensations of burning in the feet. This is usually worse at night, so the patient's sleep is often disturbed.

Foot ulcers are a very great risk in diabetics; the loss of pain sensation in the feet allows minor injuries to occur without the patients awareness. This allows infection to enter the foot, which is unable to overcome the bacteria because of an additional problem that diabetics have: poor circulation in the feet. As a result, foot ulcers may be very resistant to healing, and they often lead to amputations.

Treatment that reduces the patient's blood sugar levels to normal throughout the day will usually improve the diabetic polyneuropathy. However, this is not always the case, and also it is difficult to control diabetes in many patients. Patients have to work with their diabetologists to get their diabetes as controlled as possible if they are going to help their neurologist improve their diabetic neuropathy.

## Treatment of pain in peripheral nerve disease

Many different diseases affecting the peripheral nerves cause pain. A pinched nerve, as in CTS, often causes pain and may need surgical decompression. Pressure on a nerve root close to the spinal cord produced by a ruptured disc may require surgical removal of the disc. Treatment of the cause of a painful polyneuropathy may both relieve the pain and improve the neuropathy.

If we have no direct treatment for the neuropathy, then treatment targeted at the pain is needed. This is the situation for many patients with painful diabetic neuropathies and for those with shingles, which I will describe shortly. Nerve pains may respond to narcotics, though doctors generally worry that chronic use of these drugs will make patients dependent. Other drugs that may help suppress nerve pain are antiepileptic medications—such as gabapentin (Neurontin®), pregabalin (Lyrica®), and topiramate (Topamax®)—and anti-depressant medications like sertraline (Zoloft®) and duloxetine (Cymbalta®).

## Metabolic disorders damaging the peripheral nerves

In addition to diabetes, several other hormonal and metabolic diseases can damage the nerves. These include an underactive thyroid gland and slowly progressive loss of kidney function. Vitamins, especially the B vitamins, are crucial for nerve health. Vitamin deficiencies, particularly vitamin $B_{12}$ deficiency (also called pernicious anemia), can damage nerves. A patient I treated years ago illustrates this point.

A young woman in her twenties had gone to several doctors because of numbness in her hands and feet and weakness. Her initial doctors were not very smart. They found no neurological abnormality and concluded that her condition was "hysterical." When they later found that she had an increased level of thyroid hormone in her blood, they decided this was the explanation for her "hysteria" and began treating her for an overactive thyroid. She continued to get progressively weaker and became unable to walk. When she started to develop paranoid delusions, her doctors recommended that she be transferred to a mental hospital. At this stage, her parents decided to bring her from the city where she was then living to Boston, where she had grown up.

When I saw her she was very drowsy, with signs of spinal cord damage and a peripheral neuropathy. Simply on clinical grounds, I diagnosed vitamin $B_{12}$ deficiency, the commonest form of which is called pernicious anemia because there is usually severe anemia associated. The neurological condition, which involves damage to both the spinal cord and the peripheral nerves, is called subacute combined degeneration. We drew the necessary blood tests, particularly the tests for vitamin $B_{12}$ deficiency, and immediately started high-dose vitamin $B_{12}$ therapy. The tests showed that my patient had a very low vitamin $B_{12}$ level, as well as positive antibodies associated with pernicious anemia.

We discovered that the reason for the high thyroid hormone in her blood was that she took birth control pills (they interfere with the blood test). At that time, I did not know that vitamin $B_{12}$ deficiency produced stupor (extreme drowsiness), but when we looked up the literature of the 1930s, before the discovery of vitamin $B_{12}$ that cured the condition, we found that mental changes and stupor were well known in pernicious anemia at that time. Vitamin $B_{12}$ therapy produced a rapid recovery from almost all my patient's neurological problems, except the spinal cord damage. She remained permanently paraplegic in a wheelchair.

Peripheral nerves also need Vitamin $B_1$ (thiamine) and other B vitamins for healthy function. Peripheral polyneuropathy is quite common in chronic alcoholics who become thiamine deficient. Patients sometimes take high doses of vitamins in the belief that since a little is good, a lot must be better. However, excess quantities of some vitamins can be harmful. For example, excessively high doses of vitamins A and D may be toxic, and doses of vitamin $B_6$ (pyridoxine) in excess of 200 milligrams a day may produce a toxic peripheral neuropathy, the very condition that people are trying to prevent.

## Toxic neuropathies

Some chemicals and drugs can damage the peripheral nerves and cause a polyneuropathy. Examples include industrial toxins like triortho-cresyl phosphate, a lubricant in jet engines, and acrylamide, which is used in the building and paper industries. Thallium and arsenic, which can produce a severe neuropathy, have been used by several actual murderers as well by murder mystery writers. Most famously, the 1940s hit comedy *Arsenic and Old Lace* was a spoof on the use of arsenic as a poison.

Some chemotherapy drugs, including vincristine, cis-platinum, and taxol, may damage the peripheral nerves. Other drugs, such as colchicine (for the treatment of gout), metronidazole (Flagyl®) (for treatment of bacterial infections or to enhance radiotherapy), and some of the anti-HIV drugs, may also produce toxic polyneuropathies.

In addition to producing peripheral polyneuropathies in some patients, these chemicals have proved helpful in research into peripheral nerve disease. By understanding how each of these toxins damages the nerves, we have learned more about the biochemical processes in both healthy and diseased nerves. For instance, vincristine and colchicine break down microtubules, which are the railway lines on which the molecular motors move material along the nerves' axons. Metronidazole and the cancer chemotherapy drugs bind to the DNA and RNA of the neuron, thus inhibiting protein synthesis; this shows how important protein synthesis is to peripheral nerve function.

## Autoimmune inflammatory polyneuropathies

The immune system occasionally produces autoantibodies that cross-react with the peripheral nerves as I described earlier in discussing the Guillain-Barré syndrome (AIDP), which often develops after a bout of infectious diarrhea. More common than AIDP, which comes on over a few days to four weeks, is the more slowly developing condition called chronic inflammatory demyelinating polyneuropathy (CIDP), which is responsible for about one-third of patients with a chronic polyneuropathy. One feature of CIDP that separates it from most of the other length-dependent motor-sensory polyneuropathies is that in addition to weakness and numbness of the distal muscles of the feet and hands, patients often experience weakness of the shoulder and hip muscles.

As I described in the section on CMT disease, nerve conduction studies are very helpful in separating an axonal polyneuropathy from a demyelinating polyneuropathy. Since CIDP is mainly a demyelinating condition, nerve conduction studies assist in diagnosing the disease, since most chronic polyneuropathies are axonal in type with conduction velocities in the normal range.

Most cases of CIDP are not found to have any underlying cause, despite full investigation. It seems likely that in CIDP patients, antibodies are damaging the peripheral nerves, which usually cannot be detected. Some CIDP patients have had a recent immunization or an infection such as infectious mononucleosis, Lyme disease, or HIV. We do know that CIDP is ten times more frequent in people with diabetes than in the general population.

Frequently, we find that patients with CIDP have an abnormal spike of gamma globulin in their blood tests. We say these patients have a gammopathy. Some of these patients, including Terry, have a myeloma causing the gammopathy. These patients need treatment for the abnormal protein and for the bone marrow cancer, if one is found.

The usual treatment for CIDP is high-dose corticosteroids, such as prednisone. Unfortunately, the side effects of long-term, high-dose steroids are numerous and potentially dangerous. They include weight gain, diabetes, high blood pressure, psychological changes, stomach ulcers, thinning of the bones, weakening of the muscles, cataracts, and a tendency for relapse of infections like tuberculosis. Also, patients who take high-dose corticosteroids for long periods are at risk of collapse of their blood pressure if they suddenly stop the treatment—for example, if they forget to take their pills with them when going on vacation. The collapse occurs because chronic steroid therapy suppresses patients' adrenal glands, which help maintain blood pressure and other critical body systems. Despite the risks and side effect, patients with severe CIDP often show a dramatic response to steroid treatment.

High-dose intravenous immunoglobulin (IVIg), or less frequently plasma exchange (plasmapheresis), are also used to treat CIDP. I describe these treatments in the section on GBS, and the response can be quite dramatic in patients with CIDP.

One of my patients was a lady who had been bedridden with severe CIDP five years earlier. Since that time she had received monthly infusions of IVIg, each costing about $6,000, and she was perfectly normal clinically. In fact, she was a competitive tennis player. I came to the conclusion that she did not need the treatment because it seemed that after five years without any symptoms, the condition had gone into remission. I gradually increased the interval between infusions, with the intention of eventually stopping them. However, when the interval reached three months, she came to see me in a wheelchair because of a severe relapse of CIDP. IVIg again restored her ability to play tennis, and she eventually forgave me.

*Infections causing neuropathies*

Leprosy is caused by the only bacterial infection that directly invades the normal peripheral nervous system. The disease is caused by *Mycobacterium leprae*, the first cousin of the organism responsible for tuberculosis. This bacterium gets into the nerves and damages them. The result is loss of sensation that leads to injury and eventual amputation of fingers, feet, and even ears and nose. Leprosy also produces weakness and wasting of the muscles supplied by the infected nerves. Drug treatment, when started early, is effective but costly, particularly for patients in developing countries. A few cases of leprosy are seen every year in the United States.

Viruses are a different matter, for they often damage peripheral nerves. Shingles is a well-known condition that causes a band of painful blisters to develop around one side of the torso or down a leg or arm. The virus responsible for shingles is the same one that causes chicken pox in children: herpes zoster. After an attack of chicken pox, the virus sits hidden in the sensory ganglion neurons that lie on nerve roots. For unknown reasons the virus may break out and travel down the sensory nerves to the skin, where it produces damage, blistering, and pain. Shingles may affect the face, where it can damage the cornea and result in blindness. In perhaps 20 percent of sufferers, postherpetic neuralgia is a very painful condition that remains in the spot where the shingles blisters occurred.

Another virus that invades the sensory ganglia is herpes simplex. Herpes simplex causes both recurrent attacks of painful cold sores on the face and genital herpes.

HIV infection opened a whole new world of neurological disease when AIDS first appeared. Severe suppression of the immune system allows some organisms normally destroyed by the body's immune system to break out of control and damage the body. For example, the peripheral nervous system can be damaged by the cytomegalovirus, which rapidly produces severe nerve damage and paralysis. Also, some HIV-linked cancers, such as lymphoma, can damage the nerves, either when lymph nodes press on peripheral nerves, or when the cancer itself invades the nerves. HIV may also cause GBS, CIDP, or inflammation of the blood vessels that damages the nerves. AIDS may produce a chronic polyneuropathy, the cause of which is still unknown. Additionally, some of the anti-AIDS drugs may cause a toxic neuropathy.

# Carpal Tunnel Syndrome and Other Entrapment Neuropathies

The carpal tunnel is a narrow canal formed by the wrist bones and the tough carpal ligament in the front of the wrist. Through the tunnel run the tendons that move the fingers; the median nerve, which supplies sensation to the thumb and first three fingers; and motor fibers to the muscle at the base of the thumb. Compression of the median nerve in the carpal tunnel produces carpal tunnel syndrome (CTS).

CTS generally causes pain in the hand and is responsible for night awakening. It also produces damage to the nerve resulting in numbness of the thumb, index, and next two fingers, as well as atrophy of the muscle at the base of the thumb, which is called the abductor pollicis brevis.

Women are about three times more likely than men to suffer from CTS because their carpal tunnels are smaller in diameter. It is said that one in twenty of Americans has CTS, but if you ask people if they ever wake up in the night with their hand numb and tingling, the number is much higher.

Certain repetitive occupations, such as oyster shucking and jobs involving excessive use of keyboards and vibrating tools, predispose people to develop CTS. The economic effects of this condition are significant; the lifetime cost of medical bills and lost time for a patient with CTS is estimated to be $30,000. Repetitive occupations are particularly responsible because the repeated movements produce microinjuries to the joints and ligaments going through the carpal tunnel and hence narrow the tunnel. Certain diseases, like rheumatoid arthritis, amyloidosis (a disease in which masses of abnormal protein are laid down in the carpal ligament), and an underactive thyroid, can also lead to the development of CTS because they cause abnormal tissues to encroach upon the space in the carpal tunnel.

If the patient stops the activity that is producing the CTS, it will get better. Treatment of any medical condition causing CTS, such as giving thyroid hormone replacement if the thyroid is underactive, will also cure CTS. Most CTS patients use a brace that is designed to hold their wrist in the mid-position, between bent forward and bent backward. In this position the carpal tunnel is at its largest diameter. The brace should be worn at night for a few weeks, and the patient should avoid the repetitive work that is causing the condition.

Injections of steroids and local anesthetics into the carpal tunnel have been used to relieve the compression on the median nerve, but these injections are often painful. Surgery is usually recommended if the pain is too chronic or if there is loss of sensation or wasting of the thumb muscle that is significant to the patient. The modern treatment for severe CTS is microsurgical decompression, in which an experienced hand surgeon operates with a tiny fiberoptic camera and very small instruments inserted into the carpal tunnel through a small incision in the skin of the front of the wrist.

CTS is just one of a dozen or more syndromes that result from nerve entrapment. For example, people who repeatedly produce a forceful grip may "pinch" a branch of the radial nerve, called the posterior interosseous nerve, in the back of the forearm. This may cause pain and difficulty straightening the fingers. Surgical decompression is sometimes needed for this condition. A similar condition to CTS may affect the ulnar nerve at the elbow, but in this case surgical decompression is considerably less successful than it is for CTS.

A common entrapment is of the nerve supplying sensation to the skin along the side of the thigh. This produces a strange sensation of tingling, discomfort, or increased skin sensitivity just below the trouser pocket in a man. Patients often think that they have an insect bite in the area of hypersensitivity and are surprised to see nothing when they look at the area. This condition goes by the medical name of meralgia paresthetica. People who have lost or gained weight or bulk in their thigh muscles may develop this syndrome because the affected nerve, the lateral cutaneous nerve of the thigh, becomes kinked and pinched as it goes through the thick fibrous tissue on the thigh muscle with changes in the shape of the thigh. I have seen several people who recently started as mail carriers, walking much more than they ever have before, who have developed this condition.

## The Treatment of Peripheral Nerve Diseases

The key to the treatment of peripheral nerve disease is to find the cause. If the cause is a drug or toxin, removing the offending agent will arrest the disease and let the nerves heal. If a vitamin deficiency is at fault, vitamin replacement therapy will cure the disease. If it is possible to correct the metabolic disorder—for instance, via a kidney transplant for chronic kidney failure, or an insulin pump for a diabetic—this will improve the neuropathy. If the cause is an inflammation of the arteries going to nerves (vasculitis), treatment with high-dose steroids and perhaps cancer-treating drugs like cyclophosphamide will improve the neuropathy. If a person has a neuropathy resulting from the remote effects of a cancer elsewhere in the body (a paraneoplastic syndrome), then removing the cancer may cure the neuropathy.

In the case of the autoimmune nerve diseases, like CIDP, we have many immunosuppressant drugs. These medications can also be useful in inflammatory disorders, like sarcoidosis, where masses of inflammatory tissue form in nerves and damage them.


We neurologists have been yearning for treatments based on the discovery of nerve growth factors by Rita Levi-Montalcini, who was awarded the Nobel Prize in 1986. Nerve growth factors are natural chemicals in the body that stimulate neurons to grow. They were first demonstrated to work in laboratory studies with tissue culture, and we hoped to be able to use these "nerve fertilizers" to treat patients with polyneuropathies.

Unfortunately, nerve growth factors have not so far proved helpful to people with peripheral nerve disease because of the blood-nerve barrier. This is a special structure of blood vessel walls in nerves that excludes most toxins in the blood from reaching the nerve fibers, but also prevents the nerve growth factor proteins from reaching the neurons. What we need is for the pharmaceutical industry to make "designer" nerve growth factor molecules that will penetrate the blood-nerve barrier and be able to be taken by mouth. Such drugs might benefit hundreds of millions of patients with peripheral nerve disease worldwide.

# Sources of Further Information

## General Resources

Bloom, Floyd E., M. Flint Beal, and David J. Kupfer, eds. *The Dana Guide to Brain Health: A Practical Family Reference from Medical Experts*. New York/Washington, DC: Dana Press, 2006.

Bradley, Walter G., Robert B. Daroff, Gerald Fenichel, and Joseph Jankovic, eds. *Neurology in Clinical Practice*. 5th ed. Woburn, MA: Butterworth Heinemann, 2007.

Chapter 1:
## The Human Brain, Complex and Fascinating

Cytowic, Richard E. *Synesthesia: A Union of the Senses*. 2nd ed. Cambridge, MA: MIT Press, 2002.

Luria, A. R. *The Mind of a Mnemonist: A Little Book about a Vast Memory*. Cambridge, MA: Harvard University Press, 1987.

Ramachandran, V. S., and Sandra Blakeslee. *Phantoms in the Brain: Probing the Mysteries of the Human Mind*. New York: Harper Perennial, 1999.

Sacks, Oliver. *The Man Who Mistook His Wife for a Hat and Other Clinical Tales*. New York: Touchstone, 1998.

Sacks, Oliver. *The Island of the Colorblind*. New York: Vintage, 1998.

## Chapter 2:
# Alzheimer's Disease

Alzheimer's Association.
http://www.alz.org/index.asp.

Callone, Patricia R., Connie Kudlacek, Barbara C. Vasiloff, Janaan Manternach, and Roger A. Brumback. *A Caregiver's Guide to Alzheimer's Disease: 300 Tips for Making Life Easier.* New York: Demos Medical Publishing, 2006.

"Healthy Aging: Alzheimer's Disease." Centers for Disease Control and Prevention, September 25, 2008.
http://www.cdc.gov/aging/healthybrain/alzheimers.htm.

Mace, Nancy L., and Peter V. Rabins. *The 36-Hour Day: A Family Guide to Caring for People with Alzheimer Disease, Other Dementias, and Memory Loss in Later Life.* 4th ed. Baltimore: Johns Hopkins University Press, 2006.

"NINDS Alzheimer's Disease Information Page." National Institute of Neurological Disorders and Stroke, May 26, 2009.
http://www.ninds.nih.gov/disorders/alzheimersdisease/alzheimersdisease.htm.

Taylor, Richard. *Alzheimer's from the Inside Out.* Baltimore: Health Professions Press, 2006.

## Chapter 3:
# Stroke

American Stroke Association. http://www.strokeassociation.org.

Nadalo, Lennard A. "Carotid Artery, Stenosis." eMedicine, January 24, 2007.
http://www.emedicine.com/radio/topic133.htm.

National Stroke Association. http://www.stroke.org

"NINDS Stroke Information Page." National Institute of Neurological Disorders and Stroke, May 26, 2009.
http://www.ninds.nih.gov/disorders/stroke/stroke.htm.

Stein, Joel. *Stroke and the Family: A New Guide.* Cambridge, MA: Harvard University Press, 2004.

"Stroke." Center for Disease Control and Prevention, June 21, 2007.
http://www.cdc.gov/stroke.

Taylor, Jill Bolte. *My Stroke of Insight: A Brain Scientist's Personal Journey*. New York: Plume, 2009.

Chapter 4:
# Epilepsy

American Academy of Neurology. "Efficiency and Tolerability of the New Antiepileptic Drugs."
http://aan.com/professionals/practice/pdfs/clinician_ep_onset_e.pdf and
http://aan.com/professionals/practice/pdfs/clinician_ep_refractory_e.pdf.

American Academy of Neurology. Treatments for Refractory Epilepsy.
http://aan.com/professionals/practice/pdfs/clinician_ep_treatment_e.pdf.

Devinsky, Orrin. *Epilepsy: Patient and Family Guide*. Ohio: Cleveland Clinic Press, 2007.

"Epilepsy." Center for Disease Control and Prevention, April 1, 2009.
http://www.cdc.gov/epilepsy.

Epilepsy Foundation.
http://www.epilepsyfoundation.org.

Epilepsy Therapy Project.
http://www.epilepsy.com.

International League against Epilepsy.
http://www.epilepsy.org.

"NINDS Epilepsy Information Page." National Institute of Neurological Disorders and Stroke, May 26, 2009.
http://www.ninds.nih.gov/disorders/epilepsy/epilepsy.htm.

Wyllie, Elaine. *Epilepsy: A Cleveland Clinic Guide*. Ohio: Cleveland Clinic Press, 2007.

Chapter 5:
# Multiple Sclerosis

All about Multiple Sclerosis.
http://www.mult-sclerosis.org.

Fraser, Robert T. (ed.), George H. Kraft, Dawn M. Ehde, and Kurt L. Johnson. *The MS Workbook: Living Fully with Multiple Sclerosis*. Oakland, CA: New Harbinger Publications, 2006.

Holland, Nancy J., T. Jock Murray, and Stephen C. Reingold. *Multiple Sclerosis: A Guide for the Newly Diagnosed.* 3rd ed. New York: Demos Health, 2007.

Kalb, Rosalind C., ed. *Multiple Sclerosis: A Guide for Families.* 3rd ed. New York: Demos Medical Publishing, 2005.

Multiple Sclerosis Association of America.
http://www.msassociation.org.

Multiple Sclerosis Foundation.
http://www.msfacts.org.

"Multiple Sclerosis." National Institutes of Health, May 1, 2009.
www.nlm.nih.gov/medlineplus/multiplesclerosis.html.

National MS Society.
http://www.nationalmssociety.org.

Chapter 6:
# Parkinson's Disease and Other Movement Disorders

American Academy of Neurology. "Diagnosis and Prognosis of New Onset Parkinson Disease."
http://www.aan.com/professionals/practice/guidelines/pda/Diagnosis_PD.pdf

Dystonia Medical Research Foundation.
http://www.dystonia-foundation.org.

Graboys, Thomas, and Peter Zheutlin. *Life in the Balance: A Physician's Memoir of Life, Love, and Loss with Parkinson's Disease and Dementia.* New York: Union Square Press, 2008.

International Essential Tremor Foundation.
http://www.essentialtremor.org.

Michael J. Fox Foundation.
http://www.michaeljfox.org.

National Ataxia Foundation.
http://www.ataxia.org.

National Parkinson Foundation.
http://www.parkinson.org

"NINDS Parkinson's Disease Information Page." National Institute of Neurological Disorders and Stroke, May 26, 2009. http://www.ninds.nih.gov/disorders/parkinsons_disease/parkinsons_disease.htm

"Parkinson's Disease." MedicineNet.com. http://www.medicinenet.com/parkinsons_disease/article.htm

Tagliati, Michele, Gary Guten, and Jo Horne. *Parkinson's Disease for Dummies.* Hoboken, NJ: Wiley Publishing, 2007.

Weiner, William J., Lisa M. Shulman, and Anthony E. Lang. *Parkinson's Disease: A Complete Guide for Patients and Families.* Baltimore: Johns Hopkins University Press, 2006.

Chapter 7:
# Head Injury

American Academy of Neurology. "The Management of Concussion in Sports," 1997. http://www.aan.com/professionals/practice/guidelines/pda/Concussion_sports.pdf.

Brain Injury Association of America. http://www.biausa.org.

Bruno, Laura. If I Only Had a Brain Injury. Bloomington, IN: Xlibris, 2008.

Centers for Disease Control and Prevention. "Facts about Traumatic Brain Injury." http://www.cdc.gov/ncipc/tbi/FactSheets/Facts_About_TBI.pdf.

Multi-Society Task Force on Persistent Vegetative State. "Medical Aspects of the Persistent Vegetative State. *New England Journal of Medicine* 330 (1994): 1499–1508, 1572–79.

Jameson, Larry, and Beth Jameson. *Brain Injury Survivor's Guide: Welcome to Our World.* Parker, CO: Outskirts Press, 2007.

"NINDS Traumatic Brain Injury Information Page." National Institute of Neurological Disorders and Stroke, December 30, 2008. http://www.ninds.nih.gov/disorders/tbi/tbi.htm.

Senelick, Richard C., and Karla Dougherty. *Living with Brain Injury: A Guide for Families.* 2nd Edition. Clifton Park, NY: Delmar Cengage Learning, 2001.

Chapter 8:
# Spinal Cord Injury

Boyles, Carolyn. *A Complete Plain-English Guide to Living with a Spinal Cord Injury: Valuable Information from a Survivor*. Lincoln, NE: iUniverse, 2007.

National Spinal Cord Injury Association.
http://www.spinalcord.org.

"NINDS Spinal Cord Injury Information Page." National Institute of Neurological Disorders and Stroke, April 10, 2009.
http://www.ninds.nih.gov/disorders/sci/sci.htm.

Palmer, Sara, Kay Harris Kreigsman, and Jeffrey B. Palmer. *Spinal Cord Injury: A Guide for Living*. Baltimore: Johns Hopkins University Press, 2000.

Selzer, Michael, and Bruce Dobkin. *Spinal Cord Injury: A Guide for Patients and Families*. New York: Demos Medical Publishing, 2008.

"Spinal Cord Injury (SCI): Fact Sheet." Centers for Disease Control and Prevention: National Center for Injury Prevention and Control.
http://www.cdc.gov/ncipc/factsheets/scifacts.htm.

Chapter 9:
# The Brain and Cancer

American Brain Tumor Association.
http://www.abta.org.

Black, Peter. *Living with a Brain Tumor: Dr. Peter Black's Guide to Taking Control of Your Treatment*. New York: Henry Holt, 2006.

"Brain Tumor." National Cancer Institute.
http://www.cancer.gov/cancertopics/types/brain.

"Brain and Spinal Tumors: Hope through Research." National Institute of Neurological Disorders and Stroke, May 15, 2009.
http://www.ninds.nih.gov/disorders/brainandspinaltumors/detail_brainandspinaltumors.htm.

Davis, C, and N Tandon. "Brain Cancer." eMedicineHealth.
http://www.emedicinehealth.com/brain_cancer/article_em.htm.

Wolf, H. Charles. *Damn the Statistics, I Have a Life to Live! Coping with a Brain Tumor, My Personal Story*. Bloomington, IN: First Books Library, 2003.

Zeltzer, Paul M. *Brain Tumors: Leaving the Garden of Eden—A survival Guide to Diagnosis, Learning the Basics, Getting Organized and Finding Your Medical Team.* Encino, CA: Shilysca Press, 2004.

Chapter 10:
# Amyotrophic Lateral Sclerosis (Lou Gehrig's Disease)

Albom, Mitch. *Tuesdays with Morrie: An Old Man, a Young Man, and Life's Greatest Lesson.* New York: Random House, 1997.

ALS Association.
http://www.alsa.org.

Kessenich Center at University of Miami.
http://www.miami-als.org.

Mitsumoto, Hiroshi, ed. *Amyotrophic Lateral Sclerosis: A Guide for Patients and Families.* 3rd ed. New York: Demos Health, 2009.

Muscular Dystrophy Association.
http://www.als-mda.org.

Chapter 11:
# Migraine and Other Headaches

Buchholz, David. *Heal Your Headache: The 1-2-3 Program for Taking Charge of Your Pain.* New York: Workman, 2002.

Livingstone, Ian, and Donna Novak. *Breaking the Headache Cycle: A Proven Program for Treating and Preventing Recurring Headaches.* New York: Henry Holt, 2003.

Migraine Action Association.
http://www.migraine.org.uk.

Migraine Awareness Group.
http://www.migraines.org.

National Headache Association.
http://www.headaches.org.

"NINDS Headache Information Page." National Institute of Neurological Disorders and Stroke, April 24, 2009.
http://www.ninds.nih.gov/disorders/headache/headache.htm.

Robert, Teri. *Living Well with Migraine Disease and Headaches: What Your Doctor Doesn't Tell You … That You Need to Know.* New York: HarperCollins, 2005.

Chapter 12:
# Peripheral Neuropathies and Carpal Tunnel Syndrome

American Diabetes Association.
http://www.diabetes.org.

Ashworth, Nigel L. "Carpal Tunnel Syndrome." eMedicine, December 4, 2008.
http://www.emedicine.com/pmr/topic21.htm.

Berman, Scott I. *Coping with Peripheral Neuropathy: How to Handle Stress, Disability, Anxiety, Fatigue, Depression, Pain, and Relationships.* Lincoln, NE: iUniverse, 2007.

"Carpal Tunnel Syndrome Fact Sheet." National Institute of Neurological Disorders and Stroke, April 10, 2008.
http://www.ninds.nih.gov/disorders/carpal_tunnel/detail_carpal_tunnel.htm.

Guillain-Barré Syndrome Support Group.
http://www.gbs.org.uk.

Harrop, James S. "Nerve Entrapment Syndromes." eMedicine, December 7, 2007.
http://www.emedicine.com/med/byname/nerve-entrapment-syndromes.htm.

Latov, Norman. *Peripheral Neuropathy: When the Numbness, Weakness, and Pain Won't Stop.* New York: Demos Health, 2006.

Neuropathy Association.
http://www.neuropathy.org.

"NINDS Guillain-Barré Syndrome Information Page." National Institute of Neurological Disorders and Stroke, May 15, 2009.
http://www.ninds.nih.gov/disorders/gbs/gbs.htm

"NINDS Peripheral Neuropathy Information Page." National Institute of Neurological Disorders and Stroke, April 24, 2009.
http://www.ninds.nih.gov/disorders/peripheralneuropathy/peripheralneuropathy.htm.

Senneff, John A. *Numb Toes and Aching Soles: Coping with Peripheral Neuropathy.* San Antonio, TX: MedPress, 1999.

# Neurology 101
## How the Brain Is Put Together

I n order to grasp the essential features of neurological diseases, we
need some understanding of how the nervous system is put together
and how its various parts function.

## Anatomy of the Nervous System

The brain and spinal cord are collectively called the central nervous
system (CNS). The spinal nerves and individual nerves are called the
peripheral nervous system (PNS). The third part of the nervous system
is called the autonomic nervous system. It controls the viscera, such as
the heart and bowels, as well as the blood vessels. Sensation from these
structures also runs in the autonomic nervous system. As the name
implies, the autonomic nervous system appears to act autonomously
as it controls the functions of our heart, gastrointestinal tract, sweat
glands, and blood vessels.

The brain is comprised of several parts. The brain stem, the most
primitive part of the brain, is situated at the base of the skull at the
back of the head. It connects the rest of the brain to the spinal cord.

Through the brain stem run nerve fibers, some of which conduct information about sensation from the body toward the cerebral cortex, and some of which conduct motor messages from the cortex to the spinal cord to produce movements. The brain stem contains groups of nerve cells (neurons, see Figure 4, on page xi) that send messages to move the muscles of the eyes, face, tongue, throat, and neck. The brain stem also receives sensory messages for touch and pain felt on the face, as well as messages for hearing, coming from the inner ear, and for taste, coming from the tongue. The motor and sensory nerves of the brain stem are called the cranial nerves.

Sitting behind the brain stem is the cerebellum. This is a major center that coordinates our movements and stores memory patterns of complex motor actions.

At the top of the brain stem, deep in the center of the brain, lie the thalamus and the basal ganglia. The basal ganglia and the motor parts of the thalamus are involved in the complex coordination of movement. The sensory part of the thalamus integrates and relays sensory messages (sensory nervous impulses) from the body and head to the cerebral cortex, where they reach the level of conscious perception. Emotional responses to sensory information, particularly pain, originate in the sensory thalamus.

Below the thalamus and behind the eyes is the hypothalamus. This controls the endocrine system—the thyroid, adrenal, and reproductive glands—through the pituitary gland, which lies just below the hypothalamus. When I was doing neurosurgery I looked after an eight-year-old boy who had already gone through puberty. He was already shaving and had a deep voice because a tumor in his hypothalamus was causing overactivity of his endocrine system. The hypothalamus also contains the centers that control blood pressure, body temperature, and other parts of the autonomic nervous system. The control center for the sleep-wake cycle is also located in the hypothalamus.

The outer surface of the brain is called the cerebral cortex. This is the last area of the brain to be developed in an embryo. It is the home of the largest concentration of neurons in the body. The cerebral cortex is the location of intellect, independent thought, memory, and everything that makes us individuals. One might almost say that the cerebral cortex is where the soul lies.

The cerebral cortex consists of several lobes, each of which has a different structure and function. The occipital lobes at the back of the brain contain the visual cortex, where visual nervous impulses from the eye are perceived and interpreted. A patient who suffers a stroke in the left visual cortex is blind to the right side of the world.

In front of the visual cortex, low in the skull, lie the temporal lobes, where hearing, balance, and some of the more primitive emotions—like fear, appetite, and sexuality—are localized. Patients with seizures arising from an irritation to their temporal lobe will often have a sudden feeling of fear or rumbling in the stomach before the seizure starts. Patients with damage to the middle parts of both temporal lobes may overeat and have uncontrolled, excessive sexuality; this is called Klüver-Bucy syndrome. Patients with damage localized to the hippocampi—the medial parts of the temporal lobes—are unable to lay down new memories; this is called Korsakoff's syndrome.

In front of the occipital lobes, at the top of the skull, lie the parietal lobes. Sensory messages from the thalamus go to the sensory cortex, which lies in the frontmost part of the parietal lobes. This sensory information is then passed backward to the sensory association areas, where complex interpretation of sensations occurs. Spatial awareness is localized to the posterior parietal lobes. I have had many patients with damage to their parietal lobes who cannot find their way around their own neighborhood because they have lost all their awareness of spatial relationships, or who cannot draw the numbers on a clock face.

In front of the parietal lobes and just behind the forehead lie the frontal lobes.

The motor cortex, which is the part of the cerebral cortex that controls complex movements, is located at the back of the frontal lobes. The frontal lobes are also responsible for much of our drive and social control. I had a patient who was a pillar of society but who was arrested for sexually molesting several women on a bus and resisting arrest.

These problems led me to discover that he had a frontal lobe tumor.

There are two cerebral hemispheres, the left and the right. They are joined across the midline by a thick band of nerve fibers called the corpus callosum. The nerve fibers running through the corpus callosum are the means by which one cerebral hemisphere talks to the other. If the corpus callosum is damaged, this cross talk cannot occur, leading to conditions that are called disconnection syndromes, such as the alien hand syndrome.

The nerve fibers (axons, or "wires") running from neurons in the cerebral cortex to the deeper parts of the brain—or vice versa—make up the space between the cerebral cortex and the thalamus and basal ganglia. Because these axons are surrounded by a white, fatty covering called the myelin sheath, the area between the cerebral cortex and the deeper parts of the brain is called the deep white matter.

The brain is hollow. Its central cavities, which are called the cerebral ventricles, contain cerebrospinal fluid (CSF). The ventricles interconnect, and CSF flows from the lateral ventricles (which lie within each cerebral hemisphere) and the third ventricle (which lies in the midline of the brain) to the fourth ventricle (which lies between the cerebellum and the brain stem). CSF flows from the back of the cerebellum to the outside of the brain. It then flows over the surface of the brain in the subarachnoid space and is absorbed into the sagittal sinus—the main vein lying between the two cerebral hemispheres at the top of the brain. If there is obstruction to the flow of CSF—for instance, by a tumor blocking the flow through the outlet of the cerebellum—the ventricles become blown up and the patient has excruciating headaches.

The spinal cord runs from the back of the brain stem to the lumbar spine. Like the brain stem, it is a conduit for the sensory nerve fibers running up to the brain and the motor nerve fibers running down from the brain to control the neurons that make the muscles contract. A spinal cord injury may disconnect the arms, legs, and bladder from the brain's control; these patients may be paraplegic or quadriplegic and are incontinent.

Like the brain stem, the spinal cord has groups of motor nerve cells (motor neurons) that send messages through their axons to make the muscles contract. Sensory axons coming from the body to reach the spinal cord, as well as the motor axons going to the muscles, run together in the spinal nerves. There are pairs of spinal nerves at the level of each vertebra in the cervical (neck), thoracic, lumbar (low back), and sacral regions of the spine. Pressure on a nerve root—for instance, by a herniated intervertebral disc—is very painful and results in a pattern of nerve damage called a radiculopathy.

As the spinal nerves leave the spinal column in the cervical and lumbosacral regions, they join to form nerve plexuses that look like maps of railroad junctions. Damage to a plexus is called a plexopathy. I have cared for many patients with acute brachial plexopathy. They experience an excruciating pain in one arm that lasts for a week or more and then leads to paralysis of the arm.

Individual nerves, such as the sciatic and ulnar nerves, carry nerve fibers that make muscles contract as well as sensory fibers carrying sensory information toward the spinal cord. Motor nerves contact muscle fibers at synapses, called neuromuscular junctions. Myasthenia gravis is a disease of these synapses. Muscle fibers are designed to contract to produce force; diseases of the muscles, called myopathies, cause weakness. Most sensory fibers receive input from special sensory receptors in the skin and other organs, but pain messages often come from bare nerve endings in the skin. Damage to one nerve is called a neuropathy; damage to many nerves is called a polyneuropathy.

## Microscopic Anatomy of the Nervous System

Neurons are small cells ranging in diameter from 0.2 to 0.02 millimeter. Neurons have many projections, or branches, called dendrites. One branch is much longer than the others and is called the axon. Axons may be quite short, running only for a millimeter or so, but they may be up to a meter in length. The surfaces of neurons and dendrites are covered with nerve endings from other neurons. The contact between one of these endings and the neuron surface or its dendrite is called a synapse.

Many of the larger axons in the central and peripheral nervous systems are covered in a white, fatty myelin sheath, which is formed when the surface membrane of a supporting cell rolls around the axon. In the central nervous system, this supporting cell is called an oligodendrocyte, and in the peripheral nervous system it is called a Schwann cell. There are many millions of these cells forming chains of myelin sheaths along many of the axons of the central and peripheral nervous systems.

The human brain has about 100 billion ($10^{11}$) neurons, and the human cortex has about 0.15 quadrillion ($1.5 \times 10^{13}$) synapses. Each human cerebral cortical neuron makes contact with about ten thousand other neurons. The human cerebral cortex works like an enormously complex computer. Theoretically it can perform $2 \times 10^{16}$ calculations per second.

# Physiology of the Nervous System

The nervous system works by electricity, but it does so in a different way from the flow of electrons down a wire. The neurons and their branches are all electrically charged with an electric potential that is about -70 microvolts on the inside of the cell. This potential is maintained by a system of ion channels and pumps that transfer single charged atoms (ions) across the neuronal cell membrane from one side to the other.

When a neuron is stimulated, sodium ions flow across the membrane into the cell and short out the electrical potential (depolarize it). This stimulates the next part of the cell membrane to depolarize, and the nerve impulse spreads down the axon. Neurons occasionally fire off spontaneously because of an electrical "short" across the membrane. This can produce a brief stab of pain if it occurs in a sensory axon, a sudden twitch of a muscle if it occurs in a motor axon, or a seizure if it occurs in the brain.

The speed of nerve impulse conduction partly depends on the diameter of the axon and varies from one to sixty meters per second. The myelin sheath increases the speed of conduction along a myelinated nerve fiber. The smallest-diameter fibers in the peripheral nerves have no myelin sheaths. They are called unmyelinated fibers.

Where one neuron contacts another, they do not actually touch; there is an extremely small gap (one fiftieth of a micrometer and there are a thousand micrometers in one millimeter) that can only be seen with the help of an electron microscope. The nerve impulse leaps this gap, or synapse, by releasing a puff of a chemical, called a neurotransmitter, from the upstream nerve ending. The neurotransmitter molecules diffuse across the synaptic gap and stimulate neurotransmitter receptors on the downstream neuron. The stimulation of these receptors makes the neuron surface membrane fire off (depolarize), thereby setting off the whole cascade of the nerve impulse passing down the axon to the next neuron.

There are many different neurotransmitters in the nervous system, and each has a unique receptor on the downstream neuron. As an example, Parkinson's disease results from degeneration of dopamine-producing neurons in the substantia nigra, and it can be treated by drugs that stimulate the dopamine receptors on the neurons that are downstream from the substantia nigra.

Not all neurotransmitters stimulate the downstream neuron; some inhibit it by reacting with receptors that raise the membrane potential of the cell. The balance of excitatory and inhibitory nerve impulses affecting a neuron determines whether it will "fire" or remain "silent." In this way, the brain functions like a massive computer chip.

## Biochemistry of the Nervous System

The biochemistry of the brain is highly complex. One crucial feature is that neurons require oxygen and glucose for metabolism, and they cannot survive for more than a few minutes if their blood supply is cut off. The brain consumes about 20 percent of the total amount of oxygen and glucose used by the body, as well as 20 percent of the blood pumped by the heart, but makes up only 2 percent of the total body weight. About one-quarter of all the genes in the human genome is used only for the nervous system.

Though a few new neurons continue to be formed during life in special areas of the CNS, most of our neurons were already formed in our brains when we were born. Neurons are long-lived cells with very active DNA and RNA metabolism to synthesize the proteins for their metabolism and the constant formation of new synapses. Proteins are synthesized in the neuron cell body and exported down the axon. This is an active process requiring energy. The system is rather like a railroad. There are tracks for trains to pass up or down the nerve and engines to power those trains and to carry the goods. The whole system of trains and tracks is called axonal transport.

# Glossary

**abscess.** A focal brain infection caused by bacteria.

**absence attack.** An epileptic attack involving loss of consciousness but no convulsion.

**action potential.** The change in membrane potential underlying the passage of a nerve impulse.

**alexia.** The inability to read.

**alien hand syndrome.** A neurological condition resulting in lack of recognition of one's own hand.

**Alzheimer's disease.** A progressive dementing disease that results in plaques and tangles in the cerebral cortex.

**amaurosis fugax.** Transient loss of vision in one eye.

**amnesia.** Loss of memory function.

**amyloid.** An abnormal protein material laid down in the brain in patients with Alzheimer's disease and in other organs of the body in diseases called the amyloidoses.

**amyotrophic lateral sclerosis (ALS), also called Lou Gehrig's disease.** A progressive fatal disease resulting from degeneration of the motor neurons.

**aneurysm.** A "blowout" of a weak area on a blood vessel wall.

**angiogram.** A test that clearly shows the blood vessels.

**anosognosia.** Loss of awareness of an illness or loss of function.

**anterograde amnesia.** Loss of memories from the period after an injury.

**antidepressant.** A medication used to treat depression.

**aphasia.** Loss of language function.

**apraxia.** Loss of knowledge of how to make a complex movement.

**arteritis.** Inflammation of an artery.

**arteriovenous fistula or malformation.** An abnormal connection between an artery and a vein.

**astrocyte.** Supporting cell of the brain, one of the glial cells.

**astrocytoma.** A tumor arising from the astrocyte, one of the supporting cells of the central nervous system.

**ataxia.** Loss of accurate control of movement.

**atheroma.** Degenerative material deposited on the inside of an artery.

**athetosis.** An involuntary writhing movement.

**autoantibodies.** Antibodies produced by the body's immune system that react against the body's normal proteins.

**autoimmune disease.** A disease in which the body produces antibodies or immune cells that react against the host's own tissues.

**aura.** A phenomenon associated with and usually preceding a migraine or epileptic attack.

**autonomic nervous system.** The body system that controls the heart, bladder, bowels, sweat glands, and blood vessels.

**axon.** The longest process of a neuron.

**axonal degeneration.** Death or dying-back of an axon that results from loss of contact with or disease of the parent neuron.

**axonal transport.** A process whereby materials are conveyed along axons.

**basal ganglia.** Twin masses of neurons situated deep in the brain and involved in coordination of movement.

**beta blocker.** A medication that blocks the effect of adrenaline and is used to treat high blood pressure, angina, and migraine.

**bilevel positive airway pressure (BiPAP).** A machine that provides bilevel positive pressure breathing support for patients with failing respiration.

**biopsy.** A surgical procedure in which a piece of tissue is removed from a living patient for diagnostic purposes.

**blood-brain barrier.** A physical barrier that separates the blood from the brain and spinal cord and prevents many substances in the bloodstream from entering the central nervous system.

**botulinum toxin.** Poison produced by the bacterium that causes a form of food poisoning and is used to paralyze muscles.

**bradykinesis.** Slowness of movement seen especially in Parkinson's disease.

**brain attack.** An acute stroke.

**brain stem.** The most primitive part of the brain, situated at the base of the skull below the cerebellum.

**Broca's area.** The location of language motor function in the dominant frontal lobe of brain.

**bulbar palsy.** Paralysis of the muscles of the tongue, throat, and face, which are controlled by lower motor neurons in the brain stem (the bulb). Sometimes called progressive bulbar palsy.

**calcium channel blocker.** A medication that blocks calcium entering smooth muscle cells of blood vessels and is used to treat high blood pressure, angina, and migraine.

**callosotomy.** A surgical procedure in which the corpus callosum is cut. Sometimes called corpus callosotomy.

**central nervous system (CNS).** The brain and spinal cord.

**cerebellar degeneration.** A disease causing death of cerebellar neurons.

**cerebellum.** A major coordinating center for movement and motor memory patterns, situated above the brain stem.

**cerebral cortex.** The part of the brain nearest the surface containing the highest levels of nervous system function.

**cerebral embolus.** A blood clot plugging an artery supplying the brain.

**cerebral hemorrhage.** Bleeding into the brain.

**cerebral infarction.** Destruction of brain tissue due to blockage of an artery.

**cerebral ischemia.** Loss of blood supply to the brain.

**cerebral thrombosis.** A blockage of an artery supplying the brain.

**cerebrospinal fluid (CSF).** Fluid contained within ventricles and cerebral and spinal subarachnoid spaces.

**cerebrovascular accident.** Another term for a stroke.

**cervical spondylosis.** Degenerative arthritis of the cervical spine.

**chemotherapy.** Treatment by chemicals used to kill cancer cells.

**chorea.** A jerking, involuntary movement.

**chronic inflammatory demyelinating polyneuropathy (CIDP).** An autoimmune disease of the peripheral nerves.

**closed head injury.** A brain injury in which the skull is not penetrated.

**coma.** Unconsciousness due to damage to the brain.

**concussion.** A mild brain injury causing the patient to be confused.

**cones.** Retinal visual receptors for colors.

**conversion reaction.** Loss of a neurological function thought to be due to psychiatric causes.

**convulsion.** A seizure.

**corpus callosum.** The thick band of nerve fibers connecting one cerebral hemisphere to the other.

**corticospinal tract.** The group of nerve fibers carrying messages from the motor cortex to the motor neurons of the spinal cord.

**corticosteroids.** Medications derived from hormones secreted by the adrenal gland that, in high doses, may reduce brain swelling and suppress autoimmune diseases.

**cranial nerves.** Nerves that convey motor and sensory impulses for the head.

**craniopharyngioma.** A cystic tumor lying at the base of the brain, close to the pituitary gland.

**Creutzfeldt-Jakob disease.** A rapidly developing dementia caused by prion infection.

**CT scan.** An X-ray scan that shows thin slices of the brain.

**cyanobacteria.** Primitive photosynthetic bacteria that used to be called blue-green algae.

**déjà vu.** Feelings of familiarity; in a patient with epilepsy it is usually an epileptic aura.

**deep brain stimulation (DBS).** Stimulation of the deep parts of the brain with fine wires attached to a pacemaker under the skin.

**dementia.** Loss of the highest level of mental processes.

**demyelination.** Damage or removal of the myelin sheath of a nerve fiber.

**dendrite.** A short branch on a neuron that conducts signals to the neuron.

**denervation supersensitivity.** A phenomenon whereby neurons or muscles develop excessive sensitivity to a neurotransmitter after they lose the nerves that send them nerve impulses.

**depolarization.** A change of membrane potential associated with the passage of a nerve action potential, a wave of depolarization passing down an axon.

**diffuse Lewy body disease.** A disease with features of dementia and Parkinson's disease.

**disconnection syndrome.** A neurological condition that happens when one part of the brain gets disconnected from another, usually from damage to the corpus callosum.

**disinhibited.** The state of a patient in whom damage to the frontal lobes deprives him of his ability to control his behavior.

**dominant cerebral hemisphere.** The hemisphere in which language function is localized.

**dominant inheritance.** A disease that is inherited from an affected parent and may pass to half the children.

**dura.** The firm, fibrous covering of the brain and spinal cord.

**dyscalculia.** Loss of mathematical ability.

**dysarthria.** Slurring of speech.

**dysgraphia.** Loss of the ability to write.

**dyslexia.** Impairment or loss of the ability to read.

**dyskinesia.** An abnormality of a voluntary movement.

**dysphasia.** Difficulty producing or understanding language.

**dystonia.** An abnormal posture due to abnormal tone in muscles.

**electroencephalogram (EEG).** A study of electrical activity of the brain.

**electromyography (EMG).** A test in which recording needles are inserted into muscles to detect disease.

**embolus.** A blood clot that travels from somewhere else in the body and blocks an artery.

**emotional lability (also emotional incontinence).** Loss of emotional control due to pseudobulbar palsy.

**encephalitis.** Inflammation of the brain.

**endemic areas.** Geographic regions where a disease is especially concentrated.

**engram.** A trace of a memory in the brain.

**ependyma.** Lining of the ventricles of the brain and the central canal of the spinal cord.

**ependymoma.** A tumor arising from the cells lining the cavities of the brain and spinal cord (the ependyma).

**epidural hematoma.** A blood clot between the skull and the dura.

**epilepsy.** A disease of recurrent seizures.

**extrapyramidal pathways.** Pathways in the central nervous system that control movement without going though the corticospinal tracts.

**familial disease.** A disease that runs in families and is usually inherited.

**fasciculations.** Spontaneous twitches of small parts of a muscle, frequently seen in ALS and other diseases of lower motor neurons.

**focal seizure.** A seizure affecting only one part of the brain.

**foot drop.** The syndrome where the patient cannot lift the toes due to paralysis of the muscles at the front of the shin.

**fovea.** The central area of the retina with greatest acuity.

**Friedreich's ataxia.** An inherited disease involving degeneration of the spinal cord and cerebellum.

**frontal lobe.** The most anterior part of the cerebral cortex.

**frontotemporal dementia.** A degenerative disease affecting the frontal lobes of the cerebral cortex.

**ganglion (pl. ganglia).** A collection of neurons, such as the dorsal root ganglia that contain the sensory neurons and are located on the nerve roots next to the spinal cord.

**gastrostomy.** Insertion of a tube into the stomach through the abdominal wall as an alternative route for providing nutrition.

**glioblastoma multiforme.** The most malignant form of glioma.

**glioma.** Brain cancer originating from glial cells, the supporting cells of the brain.

**grand mal seizure.** A tonic-clonic seizure involving loss of consciousness.

**graphesthesia.** The sensory ability to recognize numbers when someone else "writes" them on the palm of the hand.

**Guillain-Barré syndrome (GBS).** The disease causing rapidly developing weakness of part or all of the body that results from autoimmune damage of the peripheral nervous system.

**hemianopia (hemianopsia).** Loss of ability to see one half of the visual field.

**hemicrania.** Migrainous headache affecting only one side of the head.

**hemiparesis.** Weakness of one side of the body.

**hemiplegia.** Paralysis of one side of the body.

**hemispherectomy.** A surgical procedure to remove all or part of one cerebral hemisphere.

**hippocampus (pl. hippocampi).** The medial part of the temporal lobe, involved in laying down new memories.

**hospice services.** A system that provides supportive medical, nursing, and other services to patients in their last weeks or months of life.

**Huntington's disease.** A familial degenerative disease involving chorea and dementia.

**hydrocephalus.** "Water on the brain" due to enlargement of the cerebral ventricles.

**hypophonia.** An abnormally soft voice.

**hypothalamus.** The part of the brain that controls the pituitary gland and endocrine system, the autonomic nervous system, and the sleep-wake cycle.

**hysteria.** An old term for conversion reaction.

**ICU psychosis.** An acute agitated confusional state that may affect a patient in an intensive care unit.

**idiopathic.** Of unknown cause.

**intervertebral disc.** A fibrocartilaginous structure lying between the bodies of two vertebrae.

**intravenous immunoglobulin (IVIg).** Purified antibodies from human blood that are used to treat autoimmune diseases.

**Jacksonian epilepsy.** Focal epilepsy spreading from the face and hand to the remainder of the body.

**jamais vu.** A sudden sensation of confusion, usually an epileptic aura.

**Korsakoff's syndrome.** A syndrome involving inability to lay down new memories.

**lacune.** A "hole" in the brain caused by stroke affecting a small artery deep in the brain.

**lateral geniculate body.** The neuronal nucleus where visual nerve impulses from the eye are relayed to visual cortex.

**lesion.** An area of damage.

**Lewy bodies.** Abnormal protein structures in neurons seen in Parkinson's disease and diffuse Lewy body disease.

**lower motor neurons.** Motoneurons in the brain stem and spinal cord; sometimes called lower motor neurons.

**lumbar puncture (also spinal tap).** A procedure in which a needle is inserted into the lumbar region of the spine to withdraw cerebrospinal fluid.

**lupus (also lupus erythematosus).** An autoimmune disease of the small-diameter blood vessels.

**magnetic resonance imaging (MRI) scan.** A scan using magnetism to show thin slices of the brain.

**masked facies.** An expressionless face seen especially in Parkinson's disease.

**membrane potential.** The electrical potential of the membrane of an excitable cell like a neuron.

**meninges.** Membranes covering the brain.

**meningioma.** A tumor arising from the meninges.

**meningitis.** Inflammation of the covering of the brain, the meninges.

**metastasis.** A mass of cancer cells that has spread from a distant source with which it is not connected.

**micrographia.** Smallness of writing seen particularly in Parkinson's disease.

**migraine.** Recurrent headaches with vascular and often neurological components.

**migraineur.** A migraine sufferer.

**mitochondria.** Microscopic structures within cells that produce most of the energy required for life of the cell.

**mononeuropathy.** A disease or injury of one nerve.

**motor neuron.** A neuron that controls movement of muscles; sometimes called motor neurons.

**motor cortex.** Part of the brain located in the posterior frontal lobe of the cerebral cortex.

**motor engram.** A trace of a motor memory in the central nervous system.

**movement disorder.** The term given to a group of neurological diseases characterized by abnormal involuntary movements.

**MS.** Multiple sclerosis.

**MS plaques.** An area of white matter (myelinated fiber) damage seen in multiple sclerosis.

**multifocal motor neuropathy.** An autoimmune disease characterized by multiple areas of damage to the peripheral nerves; this disease may simulate ALS.

**multi-infarct dementia.** Dementia caused by multiple strokes.

**myelinated nerve fiber.** A nerve fiber that has a myelin sheath.

**myelitis.** Inflammation of the spinal cord.

**myoclonus.** Shocklike contractions of muscle groups.

**myopathy.** A disease of the voluntary muscles.

**neglect.** A neurological condition characterized by loss of attention to one part of the body or environment.

**nerve conduction velocity (NCV).** The speed of conduction of nerve action potential down an axon.

**nerve conduction velocity (NCV) studies.** Electrical tests of peripheral nerve function.

**nerve entrapment.** A condition in which a nerve is pinched, as in carpal tunnel syndrome.

**nerve roots.** Bundles of nerve fibers that run from peripheral nerves to spinal cord.

**neurilemoma.** A tumor of the peripheral nerves and nerve roots that originates from the supporting cells of the nerve.

**neurofibrillary tangles.** Silver-staining structures in cortical neurons that are characteristic of Alzheimer's disease.

**neurofibroma.** A tumor of peripheral nerves and nerve roots that originates from supporting cells of the nerves.

**neuroma.** The tangle of nerve fibers that may grow from the end of a cut nerve.

**neuropathy.** Injury or disease of one or more nerves.

**neuron.** A main cell of the nervous system.

**neurotransmitter.** A chemical released at a synapse (a gap between two neurons).

**neurotransmitter receptor.** A protein that responds to a neurotransmitter.

**normal pressure hydrocephalus (NPH).** Dilation of the ventricles of brain with no obvious obstruction to the flow of cerebrospinal fluid.

**nystagmus.** Jumping or jerking of the eyes, usually due to disease of the cerebellum or brain stem.

**occipital lobe.** A region of the cerebral cortex at the back of the brain.

**oligoclonal bands.** Abnormal proteins indicating an autoimmune disease of the nervous system when present in cerebrospinal fluid.

**oligodendrocyte.** A supporting cell (glial cell) of the central nervous system that forms myelin sheaths on axons.

**oligodendroglioma.** Brain cancer that originates from oligodendrocytes.

**open head injury.** A brain injury that exposes the brain to the outside, as in a penetrating bullet wound.

**ophthalmoplegia.** Paralysis of eye movements.

**ophthalmoscope.** An instrument for examining the retina of the eye.

**optic disc.** The region of the retina where the optic nerve enters the eye.

**optic neuritis.** Loss of vision in an eye due to demyelination of the optic nerve.

**papilledema.** Swelling of the optic disc, usually caused by raised intracranial pressure.

**paraneoplastic.** A neurological condition that results from a cancer elsewhere in the body.

**parosmia.** Excessive or abnormal sensation of smell.

**paraparesis.** Weakness of the legs.

**paraplegia.** Paralysis of the legs.

**paresthesias.** Tingling sensations.

**parietal lobe.** A part of the brain situated between the frontal and occipital lobes of the cerebral cortex.

**Parkinson-plus syndrome.** A disease having features of the neurological damage seen in Parkinson's disease, but also with signs of damage to additional parts of the nervous system.

**Parkinson's disease.** A disease that results from degeneration of neurons in the substantia nigra and is characterized by tremor and rigidity.

**percutaneous endoscopic gastrostomy (PEG) tube.** A tube placed into the stomach during a gastrostomy.

**peripheral nervous system (PNS).** A body system consisting of nerve roots, plexuses, and peripheral nerves.

**peripheral neuropathy.** A disease of peripheral nerves.

**persistent vegetative state (PVS).** A syndrome resulting from severe damage to the cerebral cortex that allows reflex reactions but destroys cognitive functions.

**petit mal.** An epileptic syndrome of absence attacks in children.

**phonophobia.** A condition in which ordinary sounds hurt the ears.

**photophobia.** A condition in which ordinary-intensity light hurts the eyes.

**phrenic nerve.** A nerve from the brain stem that makes the diaphragm contract.

**pituitary gland.** The master gland of the hormonal system, lying immediately below the hypothalamus of the brain and above the nasal sinuses, which controls the endocrine system.

**plasmapheresis.** A medical procedure in which antibodies are removed from the blood by exchanging the blood plasma.

**plexopathy.** An injury or disease of a nerve plexus.

**plexus.** A complex area of interconnecting nerves, particularly the brachial plexus in the upper arm and the lumbosacral plexus in the back wall of the abdomen and pelvis.

**polyneuropathy.** A disease involving many nerves.

**posterograde amnesia.** Memory loss for a period after a head injury.

**post-LP (lumbar puncture) headache.** A headache caused by low cerebrospinal fluid pressure, which follows some lumbar punctures.

**presenile dementia.** A form of dementia commonly due to Alzheimer's disease.

**prognosis.** What is likely to happen to a patient with the passage of time.

**progressive supranuclear palsy.** The disease with progressive paralysis of eye movements due to degeneration of the connections from the cerebral cortex to the neurons in the brain stem that move the eyes.

**prosopagnosia.** Loss of ability to recognize faces.

**pseudobulbar palsy.** Dysfunction of speech and swallowing due to damage to upper motor neuron control.

**pseudo-seizure.** A condition that simulates a grand mal convulsion and is believed to have psychogenic causes.

**quadrantanopia.** Loss of ability to see one quadrant of the visual field.

**quadriparesis.** Weakness of the arms and legs.

**quadriplegia.** Paralysis of the arms and legs.

**radiculopathy.** Damage to the spinal nerve roots.

**radiotherapy.** Treatment of cancer with ionizing radiation, including X-rays.

**readiness potential.** The potential in an electroencephalogram that indicates a patient's intention to initiate a movement.

**recessive inheritance.** A disease that is inherited from unaffected parents and that may affect one-quarter of siblings.

**reflex.** An automatic response to a stimulus.

**rehabilitation.** The medical specialty committed to restoring functions of the body.

**relapse.** A new attack in a person who already has a disease, as in multiple sclerosis.

**retrograde amnesia.** Loss of memories from the period before an injury.

**rigidity.** Stiffness of limbs.

**rods.** Retinal visual receptors for black and white tones.

**root (as in sensory nerve root).** The part of the peripheral nervous system that lies within the dura and is bathed in cerebrospinal fluid.

**sagittal sinus.** The main draining vein of the cerebral cortex.

**Schwann cell.** A main supporting cell of the peripheral nervous system that forms the myelin sheath around each axon.

**schwannoma.** A tumor of the peripheral nerves and nerve roots that originates from Schwann cells.

**seizure.** An electrical "brain storm," where an epileptic discharge interferes with normal brain function and produces abnormal symptoms.

**senile dementia.** A form of dementia usually caused by Alzheimer's disease.

**sensory cortex.** Part of the brain located in the anterior parietal lobe of the cerebral cortex.

**spasticity.** Stiffness and slowness of movement of a limb due to damage to the upper motor neurons' control of the lower motor neurons.

**spasmodic torticollis.** A movement disorder where the head and neck are intermittently twisted into abnormal postures.

**spinal cord.** The part of the central nervous system running from the base of the skull to the lumbar region of the spine.

**spinal tap.** A lumbar puncture.

**sporadic disease.** A disease that occurs in a patient without any known familial or geographical cause.

**status epilepticus.** A syndrome of tonic-clonic seizures lasting for more than twenty minutes.

**stenosis.** A narrowing of an artery or other channel.

**stent.** An expandable tube inserted to keep an artery open.

**stereognosis.** The ability to tell the shape of an object, or where a digit or limb is, with the eyes closed.

**steroid.** The common medical abbreviation of corticosteroid.

**stroke.** Damage to the brain due to blockage of an artery.

**subarachnoid hemorrhage.** Bleeding into the subarachnoid space.

**subarachnoid space.** The space between surface of brain and the dura.

**subdural hematoma.** A blood clot between the dura and the surface of the brain.

**substantia nigra.** The region of the brain stem that degenerates in Parkinson's disease.

**synapse.** A connection between two neurons.

**syncope.** Sudden loss of consciousness due to drop in blood pressure; faint.

**synesthesia.** The phenomenon of perceiving two different sensations in response to only one sensory stimulus.

**temporal lobe.** The inferior part of the cerebral cortex, below the frontal and parietal lobes.

**temporal lobectomy.** A surgical procedure to remove part of the temporal lobe.

**tendon reflex.** The response of a muscle to a tap on its tendon, like a knee jerk.

**thalamus.** A body part deep in the brain that integrates and relays sensory impulses from the body and head to the cerebral cortex.

**tic douloureux.** Another name for trigeminal neuralgia.

**tonic-clonic seizure.** A seizure involving contraction and relaxation of muscles and loss of consciousness.

**tPA.** A drug used to dissolve a clot causing a stroke.

**transient global amnesia (TGA).** A spontaneous attack of confusion that resolves without treatment.

**transient ischemic attack (TIA).** An acute and transient loss of neurological function due to temporary blockage of an artery.

**tremor.** A spontaneous shaking movement, as in Parkinson's disease.

**unmyelinated nerve fiber.** A nerve fiber lacking a myelin sheath.

**upper motor neurons.** Motoneurons of the cerebral motor cortex; sometimes called motor neurons

**vasculitis.** Another name for arteritis.

**vasovagal syncope.** Transient loss of consciousness due to sudden slowing of the heart and a drop in blood pressure.

**ventricle.** A cavity of brain that contains cerebrospinal fluid.

**visual association area.** The area of the cerebral cortex, anterior to the primary visual cortex, where visual information is interpreted.

**visual cortex.** A part of the brain located in the occipital lobe of the cerebral cortex.

**Wernicke's area.** The location of language sensory function in the dominant frontal lobe of brain.

# Index

NOTE: Page numbers in *italics* indicate a graphic depiction.

# D

dacrystic epilepsy, 95
DBS (deep brain stimulation), 102–103, 138–139, 141
debulking brain tumors, 197
declarative memory, 17–18
decubitus ulcers, 178–179, 182
deep brain stimulation (DBS), 102–103, 138–139, 141
deep white matter, 278
degenerative brain diseases, 204. *See also* Alzheimer's disease; dementia; neuron degeneration
degenerative epilepsies, 103–104
delta waves in the cerebral cortex, 88
dementia
    with diffuse Lewy body disease, 142
    with Huntington's disease, 143
    from limbic encephalitis, 200
    overview, 54–57
    with Parkinson's disease, 136
    with Wilson's disease, 144
    *See also* Alzheimer's disease
demyelinating diseases
    AIDP, 242, 250–252, 260
    and axons, 110, 112, 117, 125–126, 250–251
    CMT, 254–255
    and conduction velocity, 246, 247
    and gastrointestinal infections, 251
    and nerve conduction studies, 260–261, 281
    and neurons, 111
    overview, 31, 125–126
    and trigeminal neuralgia, 234
    *See also* MS
demyelination, plaques of, 110, 117
dendrites, 46, 84, 180–181, 279–280
denervation, 246–247
denervation supersensitivity, 25–27
Depakote® (valproate), 227, 229
depression
    with ALS, 214
    antidepressant drugs, 124, 214, 227, 230, 258
    from head injuries, 170
    and MS, 124
    from spinal cord injuries, 178

from stroke of right cerebral cortex, 76
    and tension headaches, 230
Detrol® (tolterodine), 124
developmental lesions, 95
dexamethasone (steroid), 186, 199
diabetes, 54–55, 65, 261
diabetic neuropathy, 241, 244–245
diabetic polyneuropathy, 256–257
diagnoses
    of ALS, 206–207
    based on brain function knowledge, 7–8
    brain injuries, 157–159
    with knowledge of effect of various injuries, 7–8
    misdiagnoses, 78, 104–108, 114–115, 117, 258
    of MS, 113, 115
    for peripheral neuropathies, 241
    for Wilson's disease, 145
    *See also* medical tests
diagnostic neuropathy screening tests, 246
Diamox® (acetazolamide), 236
diazepam (Valium®), 148
diffuse axonal injuries, 159, 164, 170
diffuse Lewy body disease, 55–56, 142
dihydroergotamine medication, 228
Dilantin® (phenytoin), 99, 198
disconnection syndromes, 20–23
disinhibition, 10, 55
distal axon, 180
*Diving Bell and the Butterfly, The* (Bauby), 69
dizziness, 169
DNA tests for genetic mutations, 49, 143–144, 207, 245
doctor-patient relationship, 1–2, 208–209. *See also* teams of specialists
dominant inheritance, 142, 148, 205, 221, 253–256
donepezil (Aricept®), 50
dopamine, 129, 130, 131, 136–139, 281
double-blind placebo-controlled trials, 211
Down's syndrome, 39
driving
    accidents and death, 153–155, 171
    and Alzheimer's disease, 38, 40
    and epilepsy, 93, 100
    and Parkinson's disease, 137
drooling with ALS, 214
drop attacks, 91

Huntington, George, 142
Huntington's disease (HD), 142–144
hydrocephalus, 49, 57, 193, 194–195, 231
hyperactive reflexes, 12
hyperacute mononeuropathies, 249
hyperekplexia, 106
hypertension, 54–55, 65, 72, 75, 227
hypophonia, 135
hypothalamus, 16, 23, 276
hypothyroidism, 152, 245, 263
hysteria as misdiagnosis of pernicious
    anemia, 258
hysteria or conversion reaction, 108, 117, 147

# I

ibuprofen, 229
idiopathic chronic polyneuropathy, 253
idiopathic epilepsy, 86, 88–89, 91, 103
idiopathic label for conditions, 152, 243
idiot savants, 5
Imitrex® (sumatriptan), 223, 229
immune system
    antibodies, 199–202, 250–251, 260, 261
    and benign viruses, 192, 263
    and MS, 111–112, 117–118
    and polyoma virus, 122, 125
    protein formations, 116
    See also autoimmune diseases
immunizations, 118, 251, 261
immunoelectrophoresis test, 239, 245
immunofixation test, 245
immunoglobulin (IVIg), 201–202, 251,
    261–262
immunosuppression, 124, 192, 266. See
    also autoimmune diseases
immunotherapy, 201–202
Imuran® (azathioprine), 121
incontinence of urine, 52, 57, 122, 123–
    124, 182
Inderal® (propranolol), 140–141
industrial toxins, 259
infantile spinal muscular atrophy, 217
infarction, 54–55, 61, 63, 77, 226
infections
    abscesses, 11, 100, 149, 164
    cause of more serious problems versus,
        49, 54, 114
    and CIDP, 260, 261

of CSF, 162, 164
and elderly brain, 40–41
gastrointestinal, 251
headaches from, 232
leprosy, 262
meningitis, 54, 163, 164, 232
and MS relapses, 117–118
neuropathies from, 262–263
from polynoma virus, 122
seizures from, 82–83, 90–91
inflammations
    AIDP, 242, 250–252, 260
    anti-inflammatory drugs, 53–54, 97,
        228, 229
    arterial, 60, 65, 233, 245, 249, 265
    blood tests for, 208, 233
    of the brain, 133
    CIDP, 238–239, 245, 260–262
    demyelination from, 246
    encephalitis, 50, 97, 133, 197, 200
    inflammatory polyneuropathies,
        260–262
    meningitis, 54, 163, 164, 232
    and MS, 112, 116
    optic nerve damage from, 110, 112
    transverse myelitis, 186
information storage in the brain, 9–10. See
    also memory
inherited diseases
    arterial diseases, 77
    autoimmune disease tendency, 111–
        112, 113
    benign familial tremor, 140
    cerebral aneurysms, 67
    Charcot-Marie-Tooth disease, 238
    CMT disease, 238, 245, 253–255
    dominant inheritance, 142, 148, 205,
        221, 253–256
    familial ALS, 204–205, 206, 207
    familial Alzheimer's disease, 47, 49
    familial amyloid polyneuropathy, 242,
        255–256
    familial cerebellar degenerations,
        149–150
    familial epilepsy, 84, 88–89, 93–94, 98
    familial generalized dystonias, 148
    familial migraine, 221, 223
    familial Parkinson's disease, 132
    familial polyneuropathies, 253–255

# Q

# R

# S

# Other Dana Press Books
www.dana.org/news/danapressbooks

# Books for General Readers

## *Brain and Mind*

### DEEP BRAIN STIMULATION:
A New Treatment Shows Promise in the Most Difficult Cases

*Jamie Talan*

An award-winning science writer has penned the first general-audience book to explore the benefits and risks of this cutting-edge technology, which is producing promising results for a wide range of brain disorders.

Cloth• 200 pp • ISBN-13: 978-1-932594-37-9 • $25.00

### TRY TO REMEMBER: Psychiatry's Clash Over Meaning, Memory, and Mind

*Paul R. McHugh, M.D.*

Prominent psychiatrist and author Paul McHugh chronicles his battle to put right what has gone wrong in psychiatry. McHugh takes on such controversial subjects as "recovered memories," multiple personalities, and the overdiagnosis of PTSD.

Cloth • 300 pp • ISBN-13: 978-1-932594-39-3 • $25.00

### CEREBRUM 2009: Emerging Ideas in Brain Science

*Foreword by Thomas R. Insel, M.D.*

Why does mental fuzziness follow heart surgery? Can brain scans predict how you'll vote? How life-threatening is hidden brain injury? Leading scientists and writers tackle these and other challenging issues.

Paper • 188 pp • ISBN-13: 978-1-932594-44-7 • $14.95

### CEREBRUM 2008: Emerging Ideas in Brain Science

*Foreword by Carl Zimmer*

Is free will an illusion? Why must we remember the past to envision the future? How can architecture help Alzheimer's patients? This edition presents these and 10 other topics.

Paper • 225 pp • ISBN-13: 978-1-932594-33-1 • $14.95

### CEREBRUM 2007: Emerging Ideas in Brain Science

*Foreword by Bruce S. McEwen, Ph.D.*

How dangerous is adult sleepwalking? Is happiness hard-wired? Could an elephant be the next Picasso? Prominent neuroscientists and other thinkers explore a year's worth of topics.

Paper • 243 pp • ISBN-13: 978-1-932594-24-9 • $14.95

Visit Cerebrum online at www.dana.org/news/cerebrum.

## YOUR BRAIN ON CUBS: Inside the Heads of Players and Fans
*Dan Gordon, Editor*

Our brains light up with the rush that accompanies a come-from-behind win—and the crush of a disappointing loss. Brain research also offers new insight into how players become experts. Neuroscientists and science writers explore these topics and more in this intriguing look at talent and triumph on the field and our devotion in the stands.

6 illustrations.

Cloth • 150 pp • ISBN-13: 978-1-932594-28-7 • $19.95

## THE NEUROSCIENCE OF FAIR PLAY:
Why We (Usually) Follow the Golden Rule

*Donald W. Pfaff, Ph.D.*

A distinguished neuroscientist presents a rock-solid hypothesis of why humans across time and geography have such similar notions of good and bad, right and wrong.

10 illustrations.

Cloth • 234 pp • ISBN-13: 978-1-932594-27-0 • $20.95

## BEST OF THE BRAIN FROM SCIENTIFIC AMERICAN:
Mind, Matter, and Tomorrow's Brain

*Floyd E. Bloom, M.D., Editor*

Top neuroscientist Floyd E. Bloom has selected the most fascinating brain-related articles from *Scientific American* and *Scientific American Mind* since 1999 in this collection.

30 illustrations.

Cloth • 300 pp • ISBN-13: 978-1-932594-22-5 • $25.00

## MIND WARS: Brain Research and National Defense
*Jonathan D. Moreno, Ph.D.*

A leading ethicist examines national security agencies' work on defense applications of brain science, and the ethical issues to consider.

Cloth • 210 pp • ISBN-10: 1-932594-16-7 • $23.95

## THE DANA GUIDE TO BRAIN HEALTH:
A Practical Family Reference from Medical Experts (with CD-ROM)

*Floyd E. Bloom, M.D., M. Flint Beal, M.D., and David J. Kupfer, M.D., Editors*

*Foreword by William Safire*

A complete, authoritative, family-friendly guide to the brain's development, health, and disorders.

16 full-color pages and more than 200 black-and-white drawings.

Paper (with CD-ROM) • 733 pp • ISBN-10: 1-932594-10-8 • $25.00

## THE CREATING BRAIN: The Neuroscience of Genius
*Nancy C. Andreasen, M.D., Ph.D.*

A noted psychiatrist and best-selling author explores how the brain achieves creative breakthroughs, including questions such as how creative people are different and the difference between genius and intelligence.

33 illustrations/photos.

Cloth • 197 pp • ISBN-10: 1-932594-07-8 • $23.95

## THE ETHICAL BRAIN

*Michael S. Gazzaniga, Ph.D.*

Explores how the lessons of neuroscience help resolve today's ethical dilemmas, ranging from when life begins to free will and criminal responsibility.

Cloth • 201 pp • ISBN-10: 1-932594-01-9 • $25.00

## A GOOD START IN LIFE:
Understanding Your Child's Brain and Behavior from Birth to Age 6

*Norbert Herschkowitz, M.D., and Elinore Chapman Herschkowitz*

The authors show how brain development shapes a child's personality and behavior, discussing appropriate rule-setting, the child's moral sense, temperament, language, playing, aggression, impulse control, and empathy.

13 illustrations.

Cloth • 283 pp • ISBN-10: 0-309-07639-0 • $22.95
Paper (Updated with new material) • 312 pp • ISBN-10: 0-9723830-5-0 • $13.95

## BACK FROM THE BRINK:
How Crises Spur Doctors to New Discoveries about the Brain

*Edward J. Sylvester*

In two academic medical centers, Columbia's New York Presbyterian and Johns Hopkins Medical Institutions, a new breed of doctor, the neurointensivist, saves patients with life-threatening brain injuries.

16 illustrations/photos.

Cloth • 296 pp • ISBN-10: 0-9723830-4-2 • $25.00

## THE BARD ON THE BRAIN:
Understanding the Mind Through the Art of Shakespeare and the Science of Brain Imaging

*Paul M. Matthews, M.D., and Jeffrey McQuain, Ph.D.* • *Foreword by Diane Ackerman*

Explores the beauty and mystery of the human mind and the workings of the brain, following the path the Bard pointed out in 35 of the most famous speeches from his plays.

100 illustrations.

Cloth • 248 pp • ISBN-10: 0-9723830-2-6 • $35.00

## STRIKING BACK AT STROKE: A Doctor-Patient Journal

*Cleo Hutton and Louis R. Caplan, M.D.*

A personal account, with medical guidance from a leading neurologist, for anyone enduring the changes that a stroke can bring to a life, a family, and a sense of self.

15 illustrations.

Cloth • 240 pp • ISBN-10: 0-9723830-1-8 • $27.00

## UNDERSTANDING DEPRESSION:
What We Know and What You Can Do About It

*J. Raymond DePaulo, Jr., M.D., and Leslie Alan Horvitz*

*Foreword by Kay Redfield Jamison, Ph.D.*

What depression is, who gets it and why, what happens in the brain, troubles that come with the illness, and the treatments that work.

Cloth • 304 pp • ISBN-10: 0-471-39552-8 • $24.95
Paper • 296 pp • ISBN-10: 0-471-43030-7 • $14.95

## KEEP YOUR BRAIN YOUNG:
The Complete Guide to Physical and Emotional Health and Longevity

*Guy M. McKhann, M.D., and Marilyn Albert, Ph.D.*

Every aspect of aging and the brain: changes in memory, nutrition, mood, sleep, and sex, as well as the later problems in alcohol use, vision, hearing, movement, and balance.

Cloth • 304 pp • ISBN-10: 0-471-40792-5 • $24.95
Paper • 304 pp • ISBN-10: 0-471-43028-5 • $15.95

## THE END OF STRESS AS WE KNOW IT

*Bruce S. McEwen, Ph.D., with Elizabeth Norton Lasley • Foreword by Robert Sapolsky*

How brain and body work under stress and how it is possible to avoid its debilitating effects.

Cloth • 239 pp • ISBN-10: 0-309-07640-4 • $27.95
Paper • 262 pp • ISBN-10: 0-309-09121-7 • $19.95

## IN SEARCH OF THE LOST CORD:
Solving the Mystery of Spinal Cord Regeneration

*Luba Vikhanski*

The story of the scientists and science involved in the international scientific race to find ways to repair the damaged spinal cord and restore movement.

21 photos; 12 illustrations.

Cloth • 269 pp • ISBN-10: 0-309-07437-1 • $27.95

## THE SECRET LIFE OF THE BRAIN

*Richard Restak, M.D. • Foreword by David Grubin*

Companion book to the PBS series of the same name, exploring recent discoveries about the brain from infancy through old age.

Cloth • 201 pp • ISBN-10: 0-309-07435-5 • $35.00

## THE LONGEVITY STRATEGY:
How to Live to 100 Using the Brain-Body Connection

*David Mahoney and Richard Restak, M.D. • Foreword by William Safire*

Advice on the brain and aging well.

Cloth • 250 pp • ISBN-10: 0-471-24867-3 • $22.95
Paper • 272 pp • ISBN-10: 0-471-32794-8 • $14.95

STATES OF MIND: New Discoveries About How Our Brains Make Us Who We Are

*Roberta Conlan, Editor*

Adapted from the Dana/Smithsonian Associates lecture series by eight of the country's top brain scientists, including the 2000 Nobel laureate in medicine, Eric Kandel.

Cloth • 214 pp • ISBN-10: 0-471-29963-4 • $24.95

Paper • 224 pp • ISBN-10: 0-471-39973-6 • $18.95

## *The Dana Foundation Series on Neuroethics*

### DEFINING RIGHT AND WRONG IN BRAIN SCIENCE:
Essential Readings in Neuroethics

*Walter Glannon, Ph.D., Editor*

The fifth volume in The Dana Foundation Series on Neuroethics, this collection marks the five-year anniversary of the first meeting in the field of neuroethics, providing readers with the seminal writings on the past, present, and future ethical issues facing neuroscience and society.

Cloth • 350 pp • ISBN-10: 978-1-932594-25-6 • $15.95

### HARD SCIENCE, HARD CHOICES:
Facts, Ethics, and Policies Guiding Brain Science Today

*Sandra J. Ackerman, Editor*

Top scholars and scientists discuss new and complex medical and social ethics brought about by advances in neuroscience. Based on an invitational meeting co-sponsored by the Library of Congress, the National Institutes of Health, the Columbia University Center for Bioethics, and the Dana Foundation.

Paper • 152 pp • ISBN-10: 1-932594-02-7 • $12.95

### NEUROSCIENCE AND THE LAW: Brain, Mind, and the Scales of Justice

*Brent Garland, Editor. With commissioned papers by Michael S. Gazzaniga, Ph.D., and Megan S. Steven; Laurence R. Tancredi, M.D., J.D.; Henry T. Greely, J.D.; and Stephen J. Morse, J.D., Ph.D.*

How discoveries in neuroscience influence criminal and civil justice, based on an invitational meeting of 26 top neuroscientists, legal scholars, attorneys, and state and federal judges convened by the Dana Foundation and the American Association for the Advancement of Science.

Paper • 226 pp • ISBN-10: 1-032594-04-3 • $8.95

### BEYOND THERAPY: Biotechnology and the Pursuit of Happiness
A Report of the President's Council on Bioethics

*Special Foreword by Leon R. Kass, M.D., Chairman*

*Introduction by William Safire*

Can biotechnology satisfy human desires for better children, superior performance, ageless bodies, and happy souls? This report says these possibilities present us with profound ethical challenges and choices. Includes dissenting commentary by scientist members of the Council.

Paper • 376 pp • ISBN-10: 1-932594-05-1 • $10.95

NEUROETHICS: Mapping the Field. Conference Proceedings

*Steven J. Marcus, Editor*

Proceedings of the landmark 2002 conference organized by Stanford University and the University of California, San Francisco, and sponsored by the Dana Foundation, at which more than 150 neuroscientists, bioethicists, psychiatrists and psychologists, philosophers, and professors of law and public policy debated the ethical implications of neuroscience research findings.

50 illustrations.

Paper • 367 pp • ISBN-10: 0-9723830-0-X • $10.95

# Immunology

RESISTANCE: The Human Struggle Against Infection

*Norbert Gualde, M.D., translated by Steven Rendall*

Traces the histories of epidemics and the emergence or re-emergence of diseases, illustrating how new global strategies and research of the body's own weapons of immunity can work together to fight tomorrow's inevitable infectious outbreaks.

Cloth • 219 pp • ISBN-10: 1-932594-00-0 • $25.00

FATAL SEQUENCE: The Killer Within

*Kevin J. Tracey, M.D.*

An easily understood account of the spiral of sepsis, a sometimes fatal crisis that most often affects patients fighting off nonfatal illnesses or injury. Tracey puts the scientific and medical story of sepsis in the context of his battle to save a burned baby, a sensitive telling of cutting-edge science.

Cloth • 231 pp • ISBN-10: 1-932594-06-X • $23.95
Paper • 231 pp • ISBN-10: 1-932594-09-4 • $12.95

# Arts Education

A WELL-TEMPERED MIND: Using Music to Help Children Listen and Learn

*Peter Perret and Janet Fox • Foreword by Maya Angelou*

Five musicians enter elementary school classrooms, helping children learn about music and contributing to both higher enthusiasm and improved academic performance. This charming story gives us a taste of things to come in one of the newest areas of brain research: the effect of music on the brain.

12 illustrations.

Cloth • 225 pp • ISBN-10: 1-932594-03-5 • $22.95
Paper • 225 pp • ISBN-10: 1-932594-08-6 • $12.00

*Dana Press also publishes periodicals dealing with brain science, arts education, and immunology. For more information, visit www.dana.org.*